GYNECOLOGICAL ENDOSCOPY

Cover illustrations:

Upper left: laparoscopic view of the abdominal cavity showing the uterus and
fallopian tubes, ovaries and uterosacral ligaments.

Lower left: laparoscopic view showing peritoneal adhesions in endometriosis.
The bluish structure is a cyst. Part
of the uterus can be seen on the
right.

Upper right: chorionoscopic view showing a
normal villus with a large number
of syncytial sprouts. The smooth
surface of the chorion and its vessels can be seen in the background.

Lower right: hysteroscopic view showing a
normal ndocervical canal where
it app   hes the internal os,
thr   vhich the uterine fundus
i

GYNECOLOGICAL ENDOSCOPY

Alan G. Gordon MB FRCS FRCOG
Consultant Obstetrician and Gynaecologist
Princess Royal Hospital
Hull, UK

B. Victor Lewis MD FRCS FRCOG
Consultant Obstetrician and Gynaecologist
Watford General Hospital
Watford, UK

Foreword by
Patrick C. Steptoe DSc FRCS FRCOG
Director
Bourn Hall Clinic
Bourn, Cambridge, UK

J. B. Lippincott · Philadelphia

Gower Medical Publishing · London · New York

**Distributed in all countries except USA,
Canada and Japan by:**
Chapman and Hall Ltd
11 New Fetter Lane
London EC4P 4EE
UK

Distributed in Japan by:
Nankodo Co. Ltd
Tokyo International P.O. Box 5272
42-6, Hongo 3 – chome
Bunkyo-ku Tokyo 113, Japan.

Distributed in the USA and Canada by:
J. B. Lippincott Company
East Washington Square
Philadelphia, P.A. 19105
USA

ISBN: 0-397-44570-9 (Lippincott/Gower)

Library of Congress Catalog Number: 88 – 81314

Library of Congress Cataloging in Publication Data are available

Project Editor: Fiona Lake
Design: Jeremy Rose
Cover: Michael Laake
Illustration: Lynda Payne
Maurizia Merati

Typeset in Times Roman
Origination in Hong Kong by South Sea International Press
Printed in Singapore by Imago Productions (FE) PTE Limited

FOREWORD

The introduction of endoscopy into gynaecology has produced dramatic changes in clinical practice. It is gratifying that gynaecologists were the first practitioners to take advantage of the introduction of cold-light systems and the development by Professor H. Hopkins of the red lens system. No longer was the diagnosis of pelvic disease dependent on signs and symptoms, limited biochemical investigations and, often, a laparotomy of uncertain value. This frequently happened in the 1950's and 1960's. Diagnosis in gynaecology became accurate and more scientific, no longer relying on 'inspired' guesses. The safe invasion of the abdominal cavity by laparoscopy soon led to the adoption of endoscopy in other specialities.

The safety and clinical value of endoscopy favoured the development of telescopes capable of inspecting the cervical canal, the uterine cavity, the fetus in the amniotic sac and the chorionic membranes.

Many operative procedures can now be carried out safely and swiftly with little disturbance to the patient under endoscopic vision. Biopsy of tissues can be performed without undue risk. Moreover, permanent records of the pathology can be made by photography, films and videotapes in full colour.

Although ultrasonography has contributed recently to gynaecological diagnosis, laparoscopy and other endoscopies will continue to dominate for many years because of their accuracy and the fact that operative procedures are possible. As one of the pioneers of laparoscopy in gynaecology, I welcome this new well written and illustrated book by Alan Gordon and Victor Lewis.

Patrick Steptoe
Cambridge, 1988

PREFACE

In the last decade, laparoscopy has become one of the most frequently performed operations in gynaecological practice. The majority of surgeons, however, limit the use of the laparoscope to the investigation of pelvic pain or infertility. The most common and, in many cases, the only laparoscopic operation performed is sterilization.

Intra-abdominal laparoscopic surgery has progressed from simple sterilization to adhesiolysis with scissors or laser, ovarian cystectomy and destruction of deposits of endometriosis. More complicated operations, such as conservative surgery for unruptured tubal pregnancy, salpingostomy and myomectomy, demand a higher degree of skill and the use of instruments to control bleeding by heat or ligation. Professor Kurt Semm of Kiel University has been the leader in the development of these technological advances and we are grateful for his cooperation in writing the chapter on pelviscopic surgery.

Modern optics and high-powered light sources are now so efficient that the diameter of endoscopes has been reduced without loss of definition. This has allowed the development of narrow telescopes which can be inserted via a laparoscope into the ampulla of the fallopian tube. Salpingoscopy is already providing a clearer understanding of pathology in the tube. Diagnostic hysteroscopy is becoming more widely used and operative hysteroscopy is now established practice. Particular interest is being shown in the use of intratubal devices for female sterilization and laser vaporization of the endometrium in the treatment of intractable menorrhagia.

In the first chapter of this volume, the history of laparoscopy is considered in detail by the doyen of European endoscopists, Professor Hans Frangenheim. Many of the references are old and are not easily available to the reader. Apart from this, we have deliberately taken the decision to avoid references to the literature, except those relating to new techniques which are not yet well documented.

There is now such a variety of diagnostic and operative instruments that it must be confusing for the inexperienced endoscopist who wishes to equip an operating theatre. We have therefore included a chapter describing the available options and although this is by no means comprehensive, it should provide guidance in the selection of an appropriate system.

Because of the need for documentation and teaching material, we have also included a chapter on endoscopic photography. Training laparoscopists is difficult but is greatly enhanced by closed-circuit television which, although expensive, should be considered essential. Simple photographic systems are useful for teaching and also allow rare conditions to be photographed as and when they occur in day-to-day practice. Photography may also have value for medico-legal purposes, for example to confirm that a sterilization operation has been competently performed.

As it was our intention to include both standard and developing techniques, we approached many specialists in Britain and Europe; it is with pleasure that we record our thanks to our colleagues who have given us their hospitality and friendship and have allowed us unrestricted access to their slide libraries, from which this work has been compiled. We have not hesitated to express our own opinions, some of which may be controversial. We also acknowledge the contribution from Mr G I Whitehead, Ms J Sanderson and Ms R R Allburt of the Department of Medical Illustration, Hull Royal Infirmary, who photographed the instruments and scenes in the operating theatres.

Finally we would like to thank Gower Medical Publishing, and in particular Mrs Fiona Lake, for their help with the preparation of this book, and also to express our gratitude to our long-suffering wives for their constant encouragement and support.

A G Gordon
B V Lewis
Hull & Watford, 1988

ACKNOWLEDGEMENTS

The authors wish to express their appreciation for technical assistance to the following optical instrument manufacturers:

Keymed Ltd, Keymed House, Stock Road, Southend on Sea, Essex SS2 5QH, England

Olympus Optical (Europa) GmbH, Wendenstrasse 14-16, 2000 Hamburg 1, West Germany

Rimmer Brothers, 18 Aylesbury Road, Clerkenwell, London EC1R 0DD, England

Rocket of London Ltd, Imperial Way, Watford WD2 4XX, England

Karl Storz GmbH, Mittlestrasse 8, Postfach 4752, 7200 Tuttlingen, West Germany

Richard Wolf GmbH, Postfach 40, 7134 Knittlingen, West Germany

Richard Wolf UK Ltd, PO Box 47, Mitcham, Surrey, England

CONTRIBUTORS

Alain JM Audebert MD
Ancien Chef de Clinique Gynecologique
Director, Robert B. Greenblatt Institute,
Bordeaux, France

Ivo A Brosens MD, PhD
Professor of Obstetrics & Gynaecology,
Department of Obstetrics & Gynaecology,
Universitaire Zeikenhuis Gasthuisberg,
Leuven, Belgium

Michel A Cognat MD
Directeur d'Enseignement à l'Université,
Head of Department of Gynecology-
Andrology, Saint Joseph Hospital, Lyon,
France

Edgard Cornier MD
Head of Department of Obstetrics and
Gynaecology, Hôpital de Neuilly,
Neuilly sur Seine, Paris, France

Michael RM Darling MB, MAO, MRCOG
Consultant Obstetrician and Gynaecologist,
Rotunda Hospital, Dublin, Ireland

Jonathan A Davis MB, MRCOG
Consultant Obstetrician and Gynaecologist,
Stobhill Hospital, Glasgow, Scotland

Robert G Edwards DSc, PhD, FRCOG
Professor of Human Reproduction,
Cambridge University, Cambridge,
England

Hans Frangenheim Prof. Dr. med
Formerly Head of Department of
Obstetrics and Gynaecology,
Krankenanstalten, Konstanz, West
Germany

Giuseppe Ghirardini MD
Division of Obstetrics and Gynaecology,
Franchini Hospital, I-Montecchio Emilia,
RE, Italy

Alan G Gordon MB, FRCS, FRCOG
Consultant Obstetrician and Gynaecologist,
Princess Royal Hospital, Hull, England

Karl W Hancock MB, FRCOG
Senior Lecturer, Department of Obstetrics
and Gynaecology, University of Leeds,
Leeds, England

Bryan M Hibbard MD, PhD, FRCOG
Professor of Obstetrics and Gynaecology,
Welsh National School of Medicine,
Cardiff, Wales.

B Victor Lewis MD, FRCS, FRCOG
Consultant Obstetrician and Gynaecologist,
Watford General Hospital, Watford,
England

Richard J Lilford MD, PhD, MRCOG
Professor of Obstetrics and Gynaecology,
St James' University Hospital, Leeds, England

Hans-Joachim Lindemann Dr. med
Professor of Obstetrics and Gynaecology
and Head of Department, Deutsches Rotes
Kreuz und Freimaurer Krankenhaus,
Hamburg, West Germany

Joris FDE De Maeyer MD
Gynaecologist, A. Z. Saint Jozef,
Molenstraat 19, 2510 Mortsel, Belgium

Bridgett A Mason MB
Medical Director, Hallam Clinic, Hallam
Street, London, England

John L Osborne MB, MRCOG
Consultant Obstetrician and Gynaecologist,
Middlesex Hospital, London, England

Luis C Pous-Ivern MD
Director, Centro de Gineco-Obstetricia y
Reproduccion Humana, Barcelona, Spain

Ian F Russell MB, FFARCS
Consultant Anaesthetist, Princess Royal
Hospital, Hull, England

James S Scott MD, FRCS, FRCOG
Professor of Obstetrics and Gynaecology,
University of Leeds, Leeds, England

Kurt Semm O.Prof.Dr.med.Dr.med.vet.s.c.
Director, Department of Gynaecology and
Obstetrics, Christian-Albrechts-University
and Michaelis-Midwifery School, Kiel,
West Germany

Luc de Simplaere,
Chief Technician, Department of
Obstetrics & Gynaecology, Universitaire
Zeikenhuis Gasthuisberg, Leuven, Belgium

Patrick C Steptoe DSc, FRCS, FRCOG
Director, Bourn Hall Clinic, Bourn,
Cambridge, England

Christopher JG Sutton MB, MRCOG
Consultant Obstetrician and Gynaecologist,
Royal Surrey County Hospital
Guildford, England

Harry Van Der Pas MD
Gynaecologist, St. Elizabeth Ziekenhuis,
Turnhout and Academic Consultant,
University of Ghent, Belgium

John Webster MB, MRCOG
Medical Director, IVF Clinic, Park
Hospital, Nottingham, England

CONTENTS

1

HISTORY
OF ENDOSCOPY

H. FRANGENHEIM

Enormous technical advances have taken place since the idea of using reflecting light in the deeper body cavities for diagnostic purposes was first conceived, and these have led to the perfection of modern endoscopic techniques. Development was initially slow, and only in the middle years of this century have the technical problems of providing a good optical system and safe induction of pneumoperitoneum been overcome. New trocars and insufflating needles have been developed, along with safer electrical equipment and routine second puncture instruments have been introduced. Thus, it is only over the last 25 years that the indications for laparoscopy have been defined and the use of endoscopy in gynaecology advocated throughout the world.

Gynaecological laparoscopy was developed from laparoscopy used for abdominal disease by general surgeons around the early 1940s and is now routine in clinical practice. Many endoscopic techniques evolved in parallel in different countries because of difficulties in communication due to the absence of international multilingual literature and due to the presence of political constraints hindering the free exchange of scientific information. It is understandable, therefore, that from around the middle of the 1930s several developments were proceeding independently and it is somewhat difficult to place them in the correct order of priority. Many early publications do not specify whether they were reporting theoretical ideas, the results of animal experiments, or real clinical experience.

It is generally agreed, however, that it was Bozzini who first gave the impetus to endoscopic investigation in Germany in 1806. The early cystoscopes without lenses were developed by Segal in France in 1826 and Desormeaux in the USA in 1867, using light from a candle reflected into the bladder through a tube.

Nitze (1897) worked with Reinecke, a Berlin optician, and Leiter, an instrument maker from Vienna, to construct the forerunners of our present-day optical instruments. Their source of light was originally an overheated, water-cooled platinum wire, but after the invention by Edison of the electric light bulb, they combined this with their cystoscopes in 1906. Newman in Glasgow mounted an electric light bulb on the distal end of the cystoscope. In Germany, Brenner incorporated an operating channel into the cystoscope and at the same time in France, Boisseau designed an instrument with the lens separate from the operating channel. Thus, during the last century the prototypes of our modern endoscopes were perfected.

Clinical application of cystoscopy, proctoscopy, laryngoscopy and oesophagoscopy dates from the beginning of the twentieth century. From Petersburg in 1901, von Ott reported the first ventroscopies, which constituted the beginning of the 'open laparoscopy' techniques used today.

Kelling (1902) in Germany had the brilliant idea that, by filling the peritoneal cavity with air, inspection of the abdominal organs would be easier. He tried his technique on laboratory animals and called it 'coelioscopy'. Jacobaeus (1912) claimed that he was the first to apply laparoscopy clinically when he reported performing 17 laparoscopies on patients with ascites; Kelling disputed this claim. Both men should be regarded as the pioneers of modern laparoscopy.

Following these early developments, many reported case histories concerning laparoscopy were documented over a short period of time, including work by Bernheim (1911) in the USA, and Nordentoeft (1912) in Copenhagen, the latter being the inventor of the laparoscope with trocar and the first to use the Trendelenburg position. Further work was carried out by Tedesko (1912) in Vienna, Renon (1913) in France, Stolkind (1919) in Russia and many others. Orndorf designed the first triangular trocar in the USA, while in Germany, Korbsch produced a new type of insufflating needle. Unverricht (1923), also in Germany, modified the angle of vision and diameter of the lens. In Switzerland in 1925, Zollikofer recommended using carbon dioxide to insufflate the peritoneum and at the end of the 1920s, Verres of Budapest added the insufflating needle in present use to the range of equipment available.

Publications and textbooks by Unverricht (1923) in Germany, Stone (1924) in the USA and Short (1925) in England brought this further phase of laparoscopic development to a close by the end of the 1920s.

The real breakthrough for laparoscopy in the treatment of internal diseases and, more specifically, in surgery and gynaecology, occurred in the 1930s. In Germany, Kalk was given the honorary title of 'Father of Internal Laparoscopy' for his technical improvement of instruments and for his scientific work. Fervers (1933) performed the first adhesiolysis in the USA. The American surgeon, Hope, recommended replacing exploratory laparotomy by laparoscopy.

The first gynaecological reports came from Hope (1937) on the diagnosis of extrauterine pregnancy. Bösch (1936) in Switzerland suggested the use of coagulation for tubal sterilization, but it is not clear whether he had actually used this technique in practice, since sterilizations were very rare at that time. Anderson (1937) also suggested, independently from Bösch, that tubal fulguration could be performed, but it was probably Power and Barnes (1941) who were the first to actually perform the operation. That the technique of laparoscopy was developing rapidly is confirmed by the report by Ruddock (1934) in the USA, which cited 2000 cases.

In 1939 the era of culdoscopy was initiated in the USA by Te Linde, but he abandoned it soon afterwards because of the poor view of the pelvic organs in the lithotomy position. In 1942 Decker was able to achieve better results with patients in the knee–shoulder position. Culdoscopy was subsequently practised almost exclusively in the USA, apart from a few clinical trials in Europe by Palmer (1950), Thomsen (1951), Clyman (1966) and Cohen (1970).

After World War II, there was a strong trend towards endoscopy, especially in cases of sterility, led mainly by Palmer in France. Initially, he used culdoscopy with the patient in the lithotomy or Trendelenburg position, insufflating gas into the peritoneum and inserting a cannula into the uterus to mobilize it. He soon turned to laparoscopy, however, because it allowed a better view of the genital organs. His colleagues, Fourestiere, Gladu and Voulmiere (1943), invented the earliest cold light endoscope, which gave improved vision and safety.

In Germany, from 1952 onwards, Frangenheim developed a much wider field of clinical indications for laparoscopy. He modified and designed numerous instruments for laparoscopic surgery, and also made the first prototypes of the modern carbon dioxide insufflation apparatus.

Another milestone in the development of gynaecological laparoscopy was the introduction at the end of the 1950s, of electro-coagulation for tubal sterilization by Palmer in Paris and Frangenheim in Konstanz, each working independently. By 1985, this operation accounted for about 80% of all laparoscopies.

It was during the 1950s and early 1960s that the first textbooks and atlases of laparoscopy were written by Palmer (1950), Frangenheim (1959), Albano and Cittadini (1962), Steptoe (1967), Cognat (1973) and Phillips (1976).

The last and most important stage in the spread of laparoscopy around the world was the formation of laparoscopic societies. The Société Medicale Internationale Endoscopique et Radio-Camera (SMIER) should be mentioned as the oldest; others include the American Association of Gynecological Laparoscopists (AAGL) and Deutsche Gesellschaft für Endoskopie.

Jordan Phillips in the USA has made a particular contribution to the spread of laparoscopy throughout the world and has helped build its present international reputation. He formed 'teaching teams' which ran regular refresher courses, analysed current statistical information concerning laparoscopy and set up committees to study the complications of this procedure.

The latest trend, inspired by Semm in the 1970s, is to broaden the indications for laparoscopic surgery, or pelviscopy, by using new operating techniques and newly developed operating instruments. Steptoe was the first to use the laparoscope for oocyte collection prior to in vitro fertilization.

In conclusion, after more than 100 years development, it is only in the last 30 years or so that laparoscopy has achieved pre-eminence amongst all diagnostic operative techniques. In Europe at least, despite advances in ultrasonography, 20% of all gynaecological operations are now laparoscopies.

Bibliography

Albano V & Cittadini E (1962) *La Celioscopia in Ginecologia*. Palermo: Denaro.

Anderson ET (1937) Peritoneoscopy. *American Journal of Surgery*, **35**, 36.

Bernheim BM (1911) Organoscopy: cystoscopy of the abdominal cavity. *Annals of Surgery*, **53**, 764.

Bösch PF (1936) Laparoskopische Sterilisation. *Schweizerische Zeitschrift für Krankenhaus & Anstaltswesen*.

Bozzini PH (1806) Lichtleiter. Eine Erfindung zur Anschauung innerer Teile und Krankheiten. *Journal für Pracktische Heilkunde*, **24**, 107.

Clyman MJ (1966) Importance of culdoscopy in fertility studies. *New York Medical Journal,* **66,** 1867.

Cognat M (1973) *Coelioscopie Gynécologique.* Villeurbanne: Simep.

Cohen MR (1970) *Laparoscopy, Culdoscopy and Gynecolography.* Philadelphia: Saunders.

Decker A (1952) *Culdoscopy.* New York: Saunders.

Desormeaux A-J (1867) Endoscopy and its application to the diagnosis and treatment of affections of the genito-urinary passages. *Chicago Medical Journal.*

Fervers C (1933) Die Laparoskopie mit dem Cystoskop. Ein Beitrag zur Vereinfachung der Technik und zur endoskopischen Strangdurchtrennung in der Bauchhöle. *Medizinische Klinik,* **29,** 1042.

Fourestier M, Gladu & Voulmiere (1943) La péritonéoscopie. *Presse Medicale,* **5,** 46.

Frangenheim H (1959) *Die Laparoskopie und die Kuldoscopie in der Gynäkologie.* (2nd edition 1971). Stuttgart: Thieme.

Frangenheim H (1969) Coelioskopie und Douglaspunktion. In *Gynäkologie and Geburtshilfe,* Vol. I. Edited by von Käser O, Friedberg V, Ober KG, Thomsen K & Zander J. pp 875-885. Stuttgart: Thieme.

Frangenheim H (1972) *Laparoscopy and Culdoscopy in Gynaecology.* London: Butterworth.

Gunning JE (1974) The history of laparoscopy. In *Gynecological Laparoscopy: Principles and Techniques.* Edited by Phillips JM & Keith L. New York: Stratton.

Handley RS (1956) Peritoneoscopy. *British Medical Journal,* **2,** 1211.

Herstein A (1955) Culdoscopy: an adjunct in gynecological diagnosis. *American Journal of Obstetrics and Gynecology,* **69,** 240.

Hope R (1937) The differential diagnosis of ectopic gestation by peritoneoscopy. *Surgery, Gynaecology and Obstetrics,* **64,** 229.

Jacobaeus H (1912) Über Laparo- und Thoracoskopie. *Beitrage zur Klinik Tuberk,* **25,** 183.

Kalk H & Brühl W (1951) *Leitfaden der Laparoskopie und Gastroskopie.* Stuttgart: Thieme.

Kelling G (1902) Über Ösophagoskopie, Gastroskopie und Zölioskopie. *Münchener Medizinische Wochenschrift,* **44,** 21.

Klaften E (1942) In *Biologie und Pathologie des Weibes (Vol II).* Edited by Seitz L & Amreich AI. p 52. Berlin: Urban & Schwarzenberg.

Korbsch R (1957) *Lehrbuch und Atlas des Laparo- und Thorakoscopie.* München: Lehmann.

Nitze M (1897) Beobachtung- und Untersuchungsmethode für Harnröhre, Harnblase und Rectum. *Wiener Medizinische Wochenschrift,* **4,** 651.

Nordentoeft S (1912) Über Endoskopie geschlossener Kavitäten mittels meines Trokar-Endoskopes. *Verhandlungen der Deutschen Gesellschaft für Gynäkologie,* **1,** 78.

Von Ott D (1901) Die direkte Beleuchtung der Bauchhöhle, der Harnblase, des Dickdarms und des Uterus zu diagnostischen Zwecken. *Rev. Med. Tcheque, Prague,* **2,** 27.

Palmer R (1950) *La stérilité involontaire.* Paris: Masson.

Phillips JM (1976) *Laparoscopy.* Los Angeles: Williams & Wilkins.

Power FH & Barnes AC (1941) Sterilization by means of peritoneoscopic tubal fulguration: a preliminary report. *American Journal of Obstetrics and Gynecology,* **41,** 1038.

Renon L (1913) Technique et indications de la laparoscopie. *Presse Médicale,* **700.**

Ruddock JC (1937) Peritoneoscopy. *Surgery, Gynaecology and Obstetrics,* **65,** 623.

Segal HL & Watson IS (1948) Color photography through the flexible gastroscope. *Gastroenterology,* **10,** 575.

Semm K (1970) Weitere Entwicklungen in der gynäkologischen Laparoskopie-Gynäkologische Pelviskopie. In *Klinik der Frauenheilkulde und Geburtshilfe (Vol. I).* Edited by Schwalm H, Döderlein G. pp 326-339. München: Urban & Schwarzenberg.

Short R (1925) The uses of coelioscopy. *British Medical Journal,* **8,** 254.

Siegler AM (1974) Laparoscopy as a prelude to tuboplasty. In *Gynecological Laparoscopy. Principles and Techniques.* Edited by Phillips JM & Keith L. New York: Stratton.

Steptoe PC (1967) *Laparoscopy in Gynaecology.* Edinburgh: Livingstone.

Stolkind EJ (1919) The value of pleuroscopy (thoracoscopy) in the diagnosis of abdominal disease. *Medical Press.* **107,** 46.

Stone WE (1924) Intraabdominal examination by aid of the peritoneoscope. *Journal of the Kansas Medical Society,* **24,** 63.

Tedesko F (1912) Über Endoskopie des Abdomens und des Thoras. *Mitteilungen der Gesellschaft Medizinische und Kinderheilkunde (Wien),* **323.**

Te Linde RW & Rutledge FN (1948) Culdoscopy: a useful gynecological procedure. *American Journal of Obstetrics and Gynecology,* **55,** 102.

Teton JB (1950) Diagnostic culdoscopy. *American Journal of Obstetrics and Gynecology,* **60,** 665.

Thomsen K (1951) Erfahrungen und Fortschritte bei der Douglasskopie. *Geburtshilfe und Frauenheilkunde,* **11,** 587.

Unverricht W (1923) Die Thoracoskopie und Laparoskopie. *Berliner Klinische Wochenschrift,* **2,** 502.

Zollikofer R (1925) Über Laparoskopie. *Schweizerische Medizinische Wochenshrift,* **104,** 264.

CHAPTER

2

INSTRUMENTS
FOR ENDOSCOPY

The major advances in gynaecological endoscopy in the last twenty-five years have been the development of the fibreoptic cable for transmission of light and development of the rod lens, which allows a clear, undistorted view. A range of ancillary instruments has also been designed, some of which are described in this chapter, and others in later chapters when their special use is being discussed.

Gas and Light Sources

The first requirement for laparoscopy is the safe provision of a pneumoperitoneum to create space within the abdomen for examination of the viscera. The modern insufflation apparatus (Fig. 2.1) delivers gas at a constant rate while it measures the intra-abdominal pressure and compensates for leakage. Most gynaecologists use carbon dioxide, which is readily absorbed into the bloodstream and excreted through the lungs. It is safe at a rate of absorption of up to 100ml/min, but if this rate is exceeded cardiac arrhythmia can develop. Others prefer nitrous oxide, which produces less peritoneal irritation and is well absorbed, but supports combustion in the presence of methane gas, which escapes if the bowel is inadvertently punctured. Nitrous oxide may also complicate a general anaesthetic if there is intravascular absorption.

Illumination suitable for routine endoscopy is provided by a 150 watt cold-light fountain (Fig. 2.2) and transmitted to the telescope through a fibre light or liquid light cable. When using small diameter endoscopes, more powerful light sources are required and computerized flash units are needed for photography.

The gas is introduced through a Verres nee-

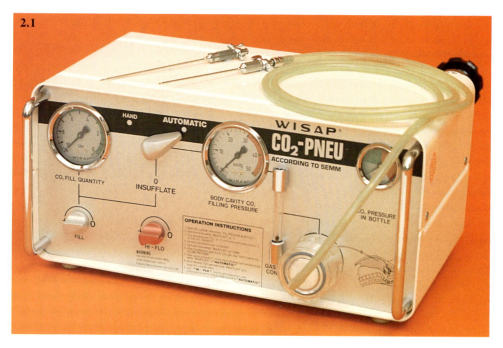

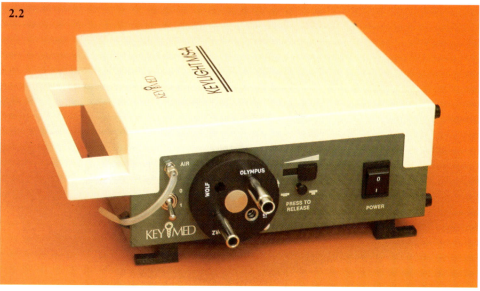

dle (Fig. 2.3). Short needles are usually safest; the longer ones are necessary only if the abdomen is very obese or if it is decided to induce the pneumoperitoneum through the posterior fornix. The needle can also be used as a palpating probe, the sharp point being withdrawn by the spring.

The choice of trocar is debatable. The pyramidal trocar (Fig. 2.4 upper) is easier to insert, but the risk of puncturing an abdominal wall vessel is greater. The conical trocar (Fig. 2.4 lower) is safer in this respect, but requires a stronger thrust to insert it.

Prior to laparoscopy for examination of the pelvic organs, it is usual to apply a cervical tenaculum to manipulate the uterus. This may have a channel for hydropertubation (Fig. 2.5 upper) or may be simple forceps with an intrauterine sound (Fig. 2.5 lower) to antevert and rotate the uterus.

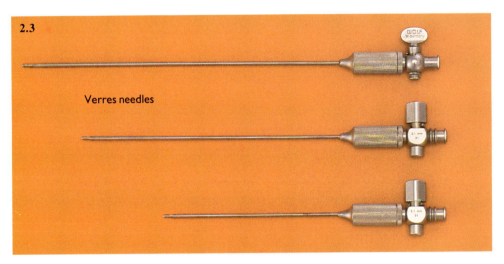

2.3

Verres needles

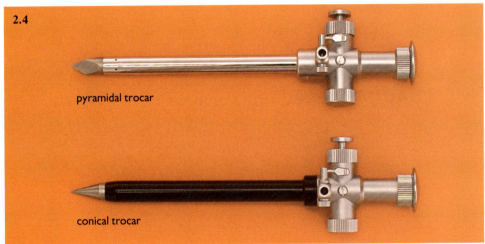

2.4

pyramidal trocar

conical trocar

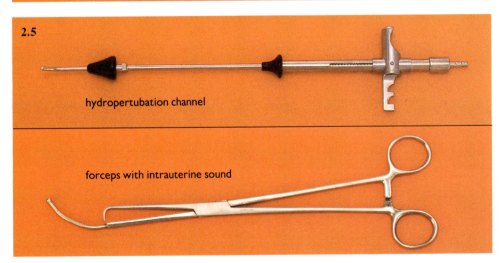

2.5

hydropertubation channel

forceps with intrauterine sound

Instruments for Laparoscopy

The development of the rod lens by Professor H. Hopkins of Reading has improved the performance of endoscopic telescopes, giving a brighter image and a wider viewing angle through a smaller diameter instrument (Fig. 2.6). Thus a modern 5mm telescope will give as good a view as the older 10mm model (Fig. 2.7), which is now required only for photography and operative work. Most gynaecologists use a 180° telescope; the 130° instrument is rarely necessary because, with the use of forceps and probes to manipulate the pelvic organs, the straight telescope provides an adequate view.

The paediatric laparoscope (Fig. 2.8) is essential for the safe examination of the prepubertal child, in whom even a 5mm telescope is too large.

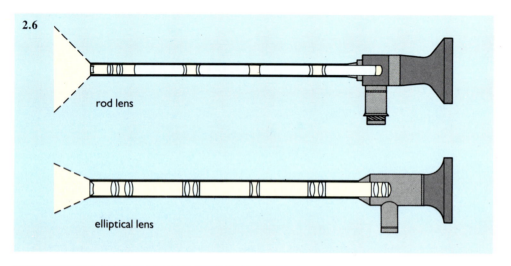

2.6

rod lens

elliptical lens

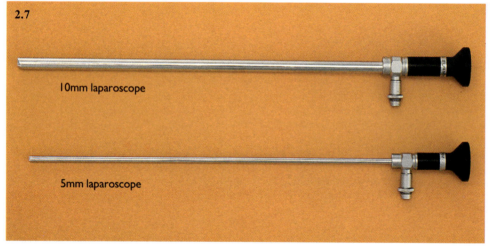

2.7

10mm laparoscope

5mm laparoscope

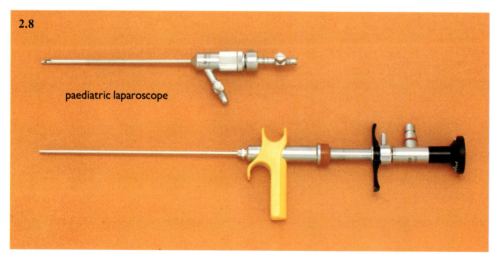

2.8

paediatric laparoscope

Operating laparoscopes are available with either an angled (Fig. 2.9) or parallel (Fig. 2.10) eyepiece. The telescope diameter is 10–11mm with a 5–6mm instrument channel. Most gynaecologists prefer to use a double puncture technique with a standard laparoscope and a second instrument, but the single puncture method is advantageous in that only one incision is necessary. On the other hand, the double puncture technique allows stereoscopic vision and therefore more accurate control of ancillary instruments (Fig. 2.11), which include atraumatic forceps, scissors and biopsy forceps. All these operating instruments are available in two lengths for single or double puncture use.

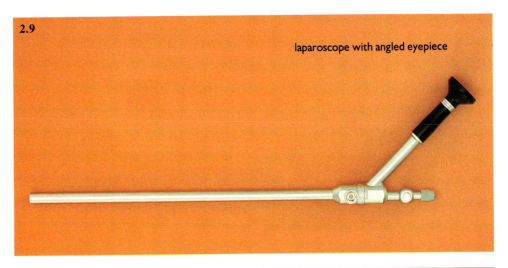

2.9 laparoscope with angled eyepiece

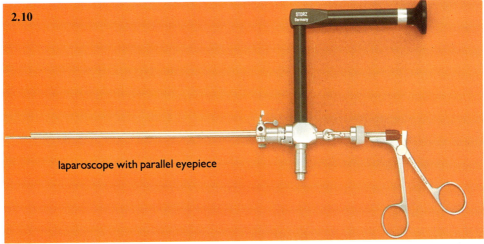

2.10 laparoscope with parallel eyepiece

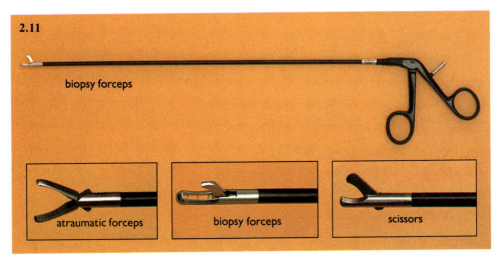

2.11 biopsy forceps

atraumatic forceps   biopsy forceps   scissors

The Semm forceps (Fig. 2.12) are preferable to forceps with scissor action for traction during pelviscopic surgery as, once applied, they do not slip off the tissues. They are used to hold the ovary during cyst resection or ovum retrieval and to retract bowel or tube during adhesiolysis.

Stronger scissors (Fig. 2.13) may be necessary if thick adhesions need to be divided or if tumours have to be resected. In the latter case, large grasping forceps (Fig. 2.14) replace the fine atraumatic forceps normally used.

Gentle traction is aided by the suction manipulator, by which the fallopian tubes can be lifted using the suction power applied by a 10ml syringe (Fig.2.15). The bowel, appendix or ovary can also be manipulated without damage.

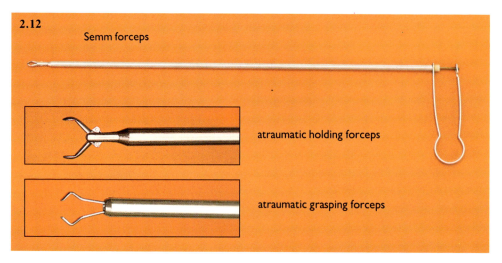

2.12

Semm forceps

atraumatic holding forceps

atraumatic grasping forceps

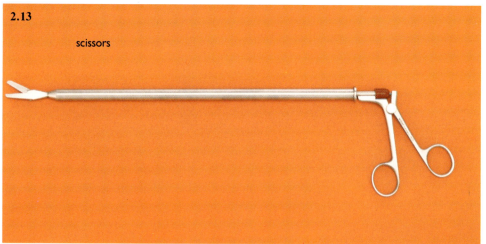

2.13

scissors

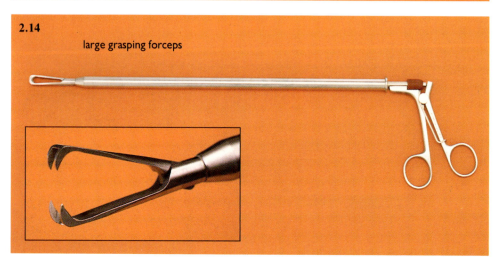

2.14

large grasping forceps

The cannula is also used for peritoneal lavage to wash out blood in pelviscopic surgery.

Palmer biopsy forceps (Fig. 2.16) were formerly the most frequently used ancillary instrument for unipolar tubal electrocoagulation and ovarian biopsy. These forceps are traumatic and the unipolar current is potentially dangerous because excessive heat is produced.

Also, the electrical current must return along the surface of bowel to reach the external electrode, thus introducing a risk of electrical burns. If electrocoagulation is used, bipolar forceps (Fig. 2.17) are safer because the current passes directly from one blade to the other and there is less danger of burns occurring outside the visual field of the surgeon.

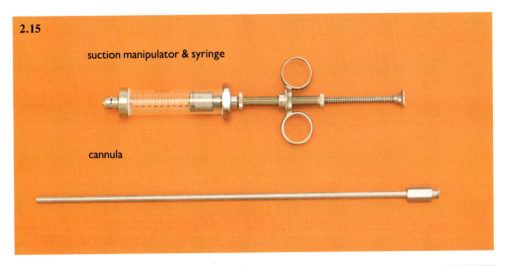

2.15

suction manipulator & syringe

cannula

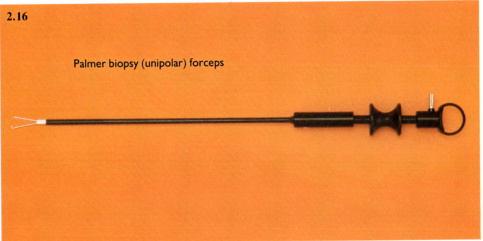

2.16

Palmer biopsy (unipolar) forceps

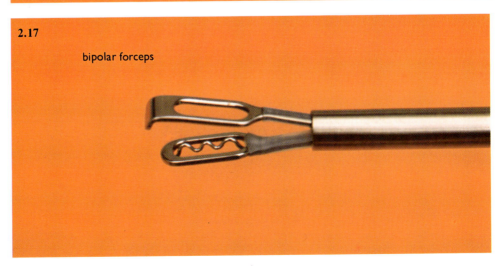

2.17

bipolar forceps

A safer form of coagulation is provided by the Endocoagulator (Fig. 2.18), which uses a current of only 5 volts. The tissues grasped between the blades of crocodile forceps (Fig. 2.19) are heated to a preselected temperature of 110–140°C for 20–30 seconds. The Endocoagulator has a dial indicating the operating temperature and an acoustic signal allows the surgeon to be aware that the instrument is functioning without lifting his eye from the endoscope. The heat is transmitted to the tissues either by crocodile forceps or a point coagulator (Fig. 2.20) and allows safe coagulation of adhesions and endometriosis and the control of intraperitoneal bleeding.

Instruments for Hysteroscopy

The hysteroscope is a modified cystoscope with an insufflating channel to deliver gas or fluid into the uterine cavity.

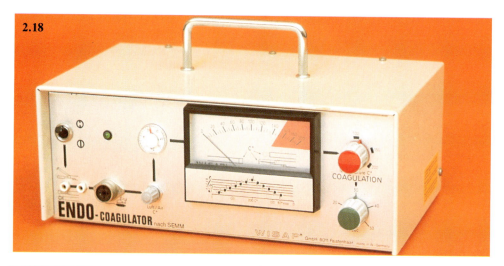

2.18

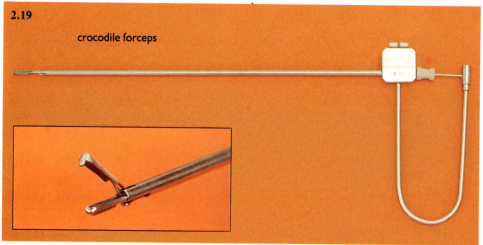

2.19

crocodile forceps

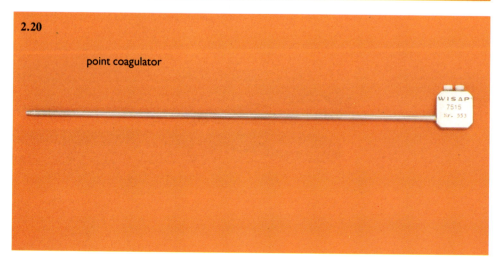

2.20

point coagulator

If carbon dioxide is used to distend the uterus, the Metromat (Fig. 2.21) or Hysteroflator with a maximal flow rate of 100ml/min at low pressure must be used, as the pneumoperitoneum apparatus for laparoscopy is unsafe for this purpose. The 4mm telescope can be combined with a 7mm operating sheath (Fig. 2.22) for probes, biopsy forceps or scissors. These are necessarily of small size, usually about 5–7Fr (Fig.2.23), which limits their strength and value, although diathermy and recently laser are increasing the scope of intrauterine surgery.

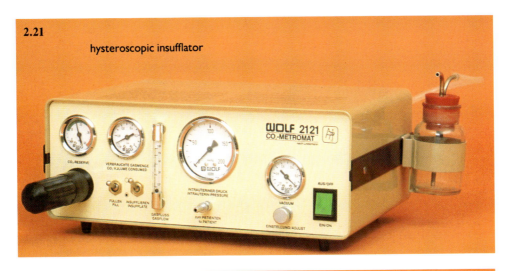

2.21 hysteroscopic insufflator

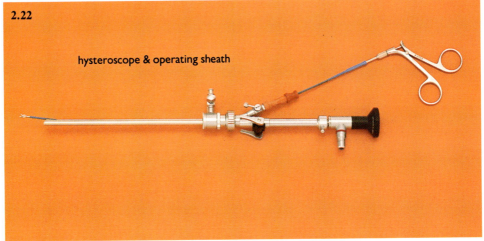

2.22 hysteroscope & operating sheath

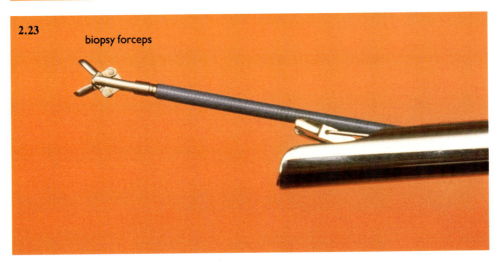

2.23 biopsy forceps

Flexible endoscopy using a 3–5mm directional endoscope with an insufflating channel is now under trial and is proving useful in both hysteroscopy and salpingoscopy. The latest endoscopes from Olympus are 3.4mm in diameter and are easily inserted into the uterus and tubal ampulla. The larger endoscopes have a channel wide enough to accommodate scissors and biopsy forceps (Fig.2.24).

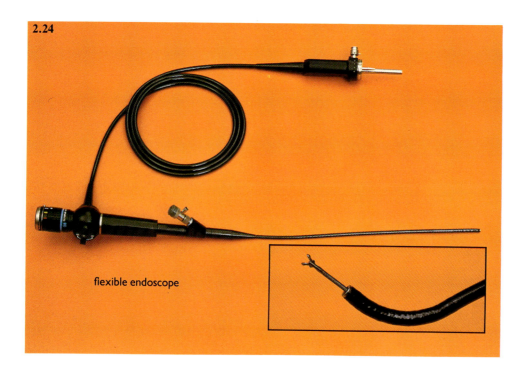

2.24

flexible endoscope

3

LAPAROSCOPY

Introduction

Laparoscopy is an operative procedure which should be performed by an experienced surgeon who is competent to deal with any complications which might arise. An assistant and a full team of nurses should be present, and junior doctors in training must be adequately supervised until their technique is perfect.

Technique

The patient is anaesthetized using muscle relaxants, endotracheal intubation and positive pressure respiration. Throughout the operation, the anaesthetist continually monitors the patient's heart rate and blood pressure.

She is placed in a modified lithotomy position (Fig. 3.1), with her legs flexed to 45° and a Trendelenburg tilt of 15°. A steeper tilt may be necessary if loops of bowel prevent easy access to the pelvis. The patient's buttocks protrude over the end of the operating table, which should have a non-slip mattress.

The theatre nurse should have available the basic laparoscopic instruments, as well as additional instruments for immediate laparotomy.

A teaching aid or closed-circuit television is invaluable for instructing staff in training; it also enables assistants to hold instruments and retract tissues.

The surgeon cleanses the abdomen with a suitable antiseptic solution, paying particular attention to the umbilicus. The assistant cleanses the vulva and vagina, ensures that the bladder is empty and applies a cervical tenaculum to manipulate the uterus and give the surgeon an adequate view of the pelvis. After testing the patency of the Verres needle, the surgeon prepares to insert it through the umbilicus with the right hand, while holding up the abdominal wall with the left hand to lift it away from the underlying viscera and blood vessels (Fig.3.2). The insertion should be through the deepest part of the umbilicus, because at this point the thickness of the abdominal wall is minimal and the peritoneum is closely adherent to the underlying tissues, making it less likely to peel off and produce an extraperitoneal gas insufflation. The position of the needle within the peritoneum is checked by the aspiration test (Fig. 3.3). Normal saline is injected through the needle and is then aspirated. If the needle lies in the peritoneal cavity, no fluid is withdrawn because it will have become distributed between loops of bowel. If the needle lies in the abdominal wall clear fluid is withdrawn, but if it is in bowel or a blood vessel the aspirate will be stained brown or red; the surgeon must then decide whether or not to proceed with the laparoscopy.

The standard method of transumbilical insertion of the Verres needle may not be possible if the patient is very obese or has a significant amount of abdominal wall scar tissue. In the latter case, the pneumoperitoneum can be introduced through the posterior fornix using a tenaculum which pulls the cervix forwards to stretch the uterosacral ligaments and put the

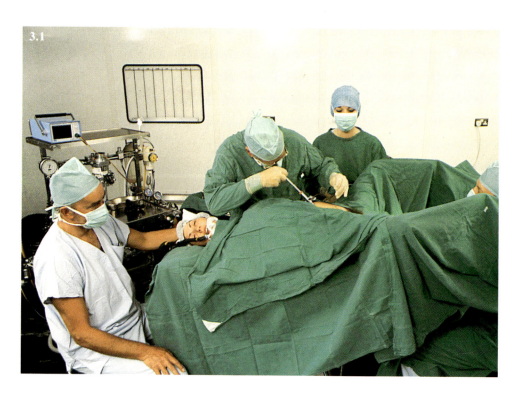

3.2

floor of the pouch of Douglas under tension. In Fig.3.4 the needle has been left *in situ* while the pouch of Douglas is inspected through the laparoscope for damage to bowel or vessels.

The pneumoperitoneum is produced by insufflating 1–2 litres of carbon dioxide, although more may be needed in the obese patient. When the gas is flowing freely and the intra-

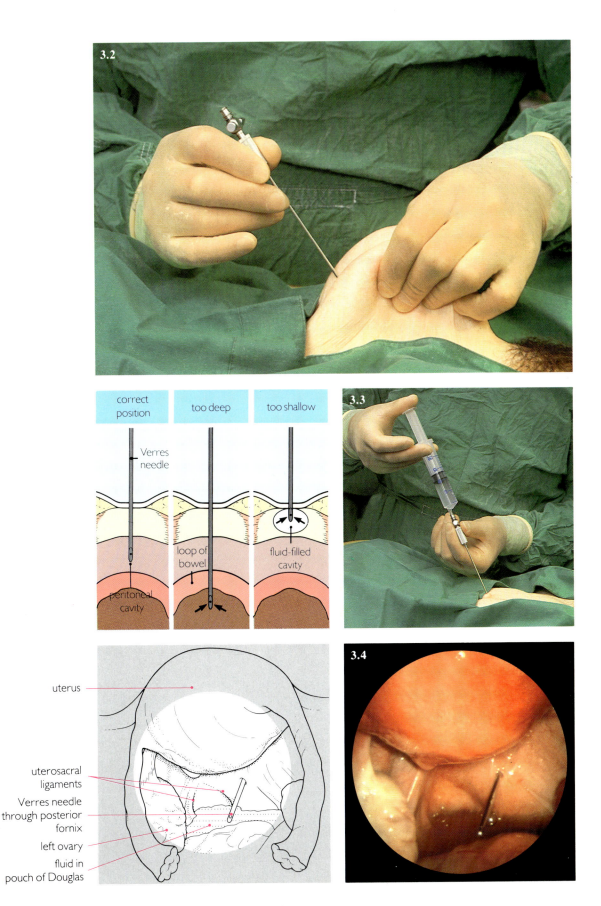

abominal pressure is normal, the rate of flow can be increased to 3 litres/min. Before inserting the trocar, the space produced by the gas is explored with a needle (Fig.3.5). If gas cannot be withdrawn freely after probing in several directions, adhesions of bowel or omentum are probably present and insertion of the trocar could cause damage.

An incision of 0.5–1.0cm in length, depending on the diameter of the laparoscope, is made downwards from the deepest point of the umbilicus and the trocar is inserted using steady pressure and directing it in a zig-zag path to prevent herniation of omentum (Fig.3.6). The abdominal wall is held up with the other hand to avoid damage to the bowel by the trocar (Fig.3.7).

A warmed telescope is now inserted and the abdominal cavity inspected (Fig.3.8). It is always necessary to insert a second instrument;

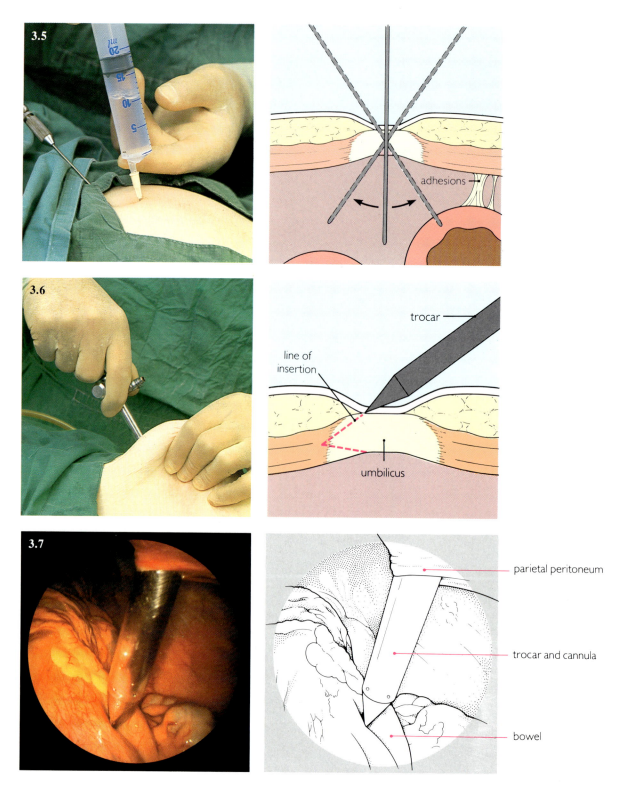

this should be done under direct vision when the trocar is seen to tent the peritoneum (Fig.3.9), before puncturing it. The second instrument may be a long Verres needle, atraumatic forceps or a simple probe (Fig.3.10), which is used to mobilize organs to obtain a better view.

The second instrument can be inserted suprapubically in the midline, or more laterally.

The abdominal wall must be transilluminted to avoid damage to an artery and if a lateral insertion is employed, the trocar should be angled medially to prevent damage to the iliac vessels. A pyramidal trocar is easier to insert than a conical one, but the former does carry more risk of puncturing vessels and causing bleeding into the abdominal wall.

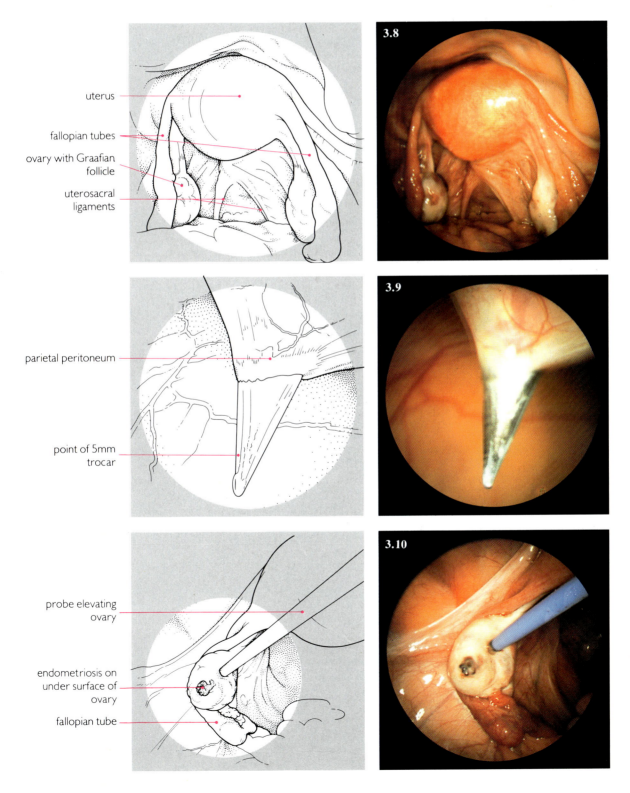

uterus

fallopian tubes

ovary with Graafian follicle

uterosacral ligaments

3.8

parietal peritoneum

point of 5mm trocar

3.9

probe elevating ovary

endometriosis on under surface of ovary

fallopian tube

3.10

Inspection of the pelvis

The surgeon first examines the anterior surface of the uterus, which is then anteverted to bring the posterior surface, uterosacral ligaments and the pouch of Douglas into view (Fig.3.11). Normally, the pouch contains up to 50ml of serous fluid (Figs.3.12 & 3.13) which can be aspirated for cytology and culture.

When the panoramic inspection has been completed, a more detailed examination is made by advancing the telescope deeper into the pouch of Douglas to examine the uterosacral ligaments and the pelvic peritoneum, where spots of endometriosis are frequently found. Small deposits may not be detected unless a close-up view is obtained.

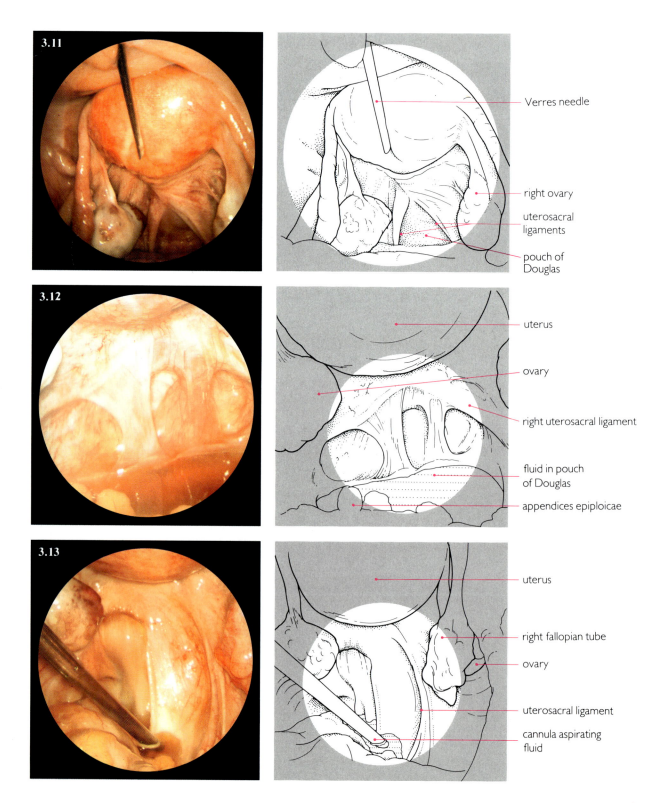

3.11 — Verres needle — right ovary — uterosacral ligaments — pouch of Douglas

3.12 — uterus — ovary — right uterosacral ligament — fluid in pouch of Douglas — appendices epiploicae

3.13 — uterus — right fallopian tube — ovary — uterosacral ligament — cannula aspirating fluid

The examination should be systematic, beginning with the ovary. The medial side is inspected closely. Depending on the time in the cycle, evidence of ovulation may be seen (Fig.3.14). It is usually easier to lift the ovary by placing the probe under the ovarian ligament and rolling the ovary upwards (Fig.3.15), but occasionally it is more easily lifted by a probe under the ovaricopelvic ligament. In this way, a follicular cyst or corpus luteum on the lateral side will be seen, and spots of endometriosis or adhesions will not be missed. In the case shown in Fig.3.16, this simple manoeuvre detected fine adhesions between the ovary and broad ligament, enabling the diagnosis and treatment of a possible cause of infertility.

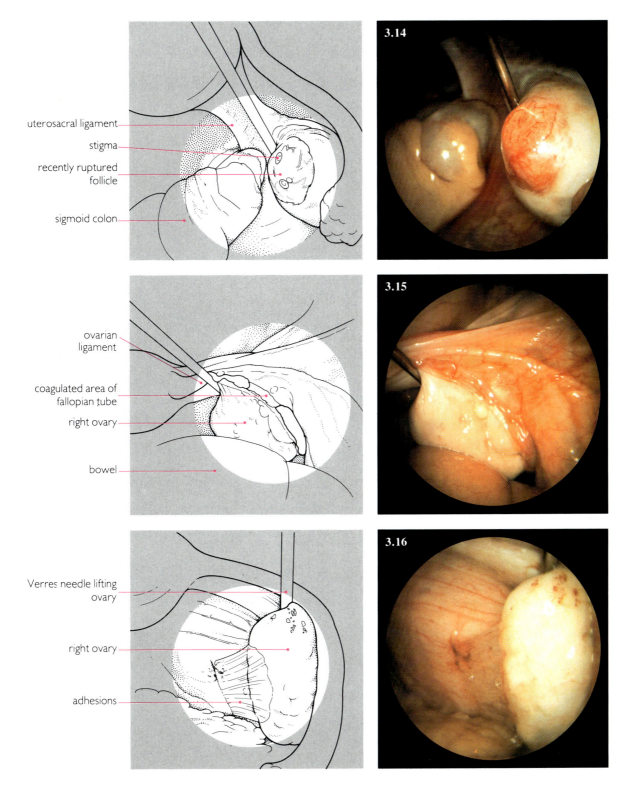

The full length of the fallopian tube must be visible so that the fimbriae can be inspected (Fig.3.17); this is achieved by lifting the tube with a probe. The procedure tends to be more difficult on the left side, where the sigmoid colon obscures the view and is often adherent to the round ligament, limiting access to the tube and ovary. A slightly steeper Trendelenburg position and careful manipulation of the tube and bowel with atraumatic forceps should always expose the fimbriae. A fimbrial cyst (Fig.3.18) or a hydatid of Morgagni are common findings.

Insertion of the telescope deeper into the pelvis gives a close-up view of the pouch and uterosacral ligaments (Fig.3.19).

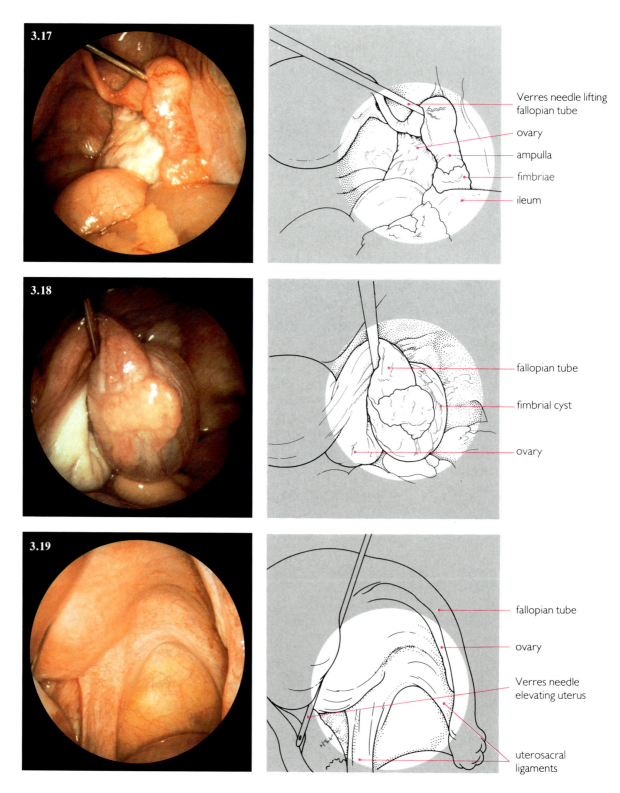

3.17
Verres needle lifting fallopian tube
ovary
ampulla
fimbriae
ileum

3.18
fallopian tube
fimbrial cyst
ovary

3.19
fallopian tube
ovary
Verres needle elevating uterus
uterosacral ligaments

Inspection of the abdomen

The external iliac artery lies in the pelvic side wall (Fig.3.20) and must be avoided when inserting the second instrument if this is positioned laterally. It is always necessary to direct the point medially to avoid it. The appendix is visible on the right side (Fig.3.21); if it is retrocaecal in position, only the base may be seen. If bowel is overlying the appendix, traction with forceps will usually bring it into view unless the tip is tied down by adhesions.

Although the gynaecologist is primarily concerned with the pelvic organs, the rest of the abdominal cavity must be routinely examined. The surface of bowel should be inspected and a probe used to palpate the consistency if malignancy or diverticular disease is suspected. Examination of the gallbladder, the superior surface of the liver and undersurface of the diaphragm complete the examination (Fig.3.22). The splenic and hepatic flexures are usually inaccessible.

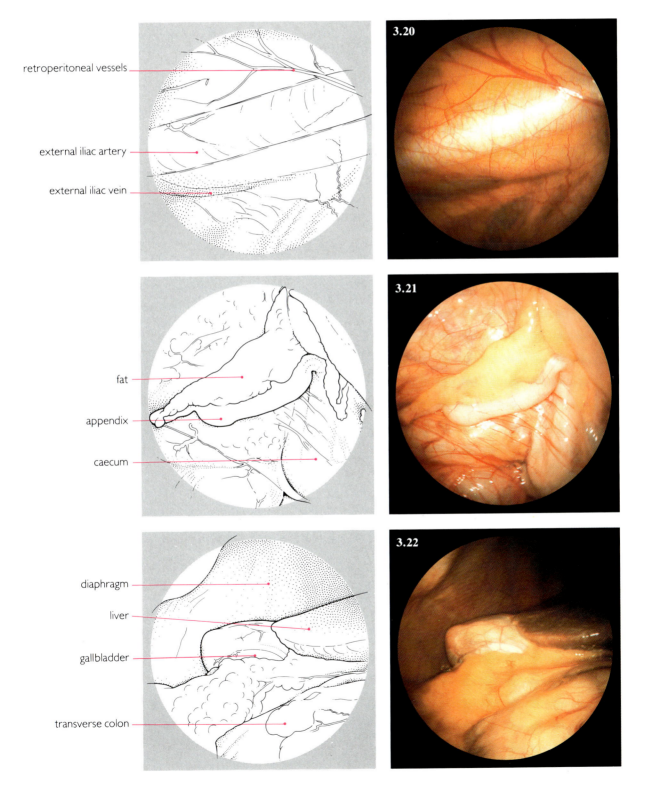

retroperitoneal vessels

external iliac artery

external iliac vein

3.20

fat

appendix

caecum

3.21

diaphragm

liver

gallbladder

transverse colon

3.22

Occasionally, it is necessary to perform laparoscopy on a child using a paediatric laparoscope (Fig.3.23); it is therefore important to recognize the normal prepubertal pelvis. The uterus (Fig.3.24) is small, measuring about 2cm in length. The ovaries (Fig.3.25) are also small, pearly white and smooth, with no developing follicles.

It is much more dangerous to perform laparoscopy in a child because the small abdominal cavity increases the risk of damage to viscera and vessels, thus the procedure should be performed only by an experienced laparoscopist.

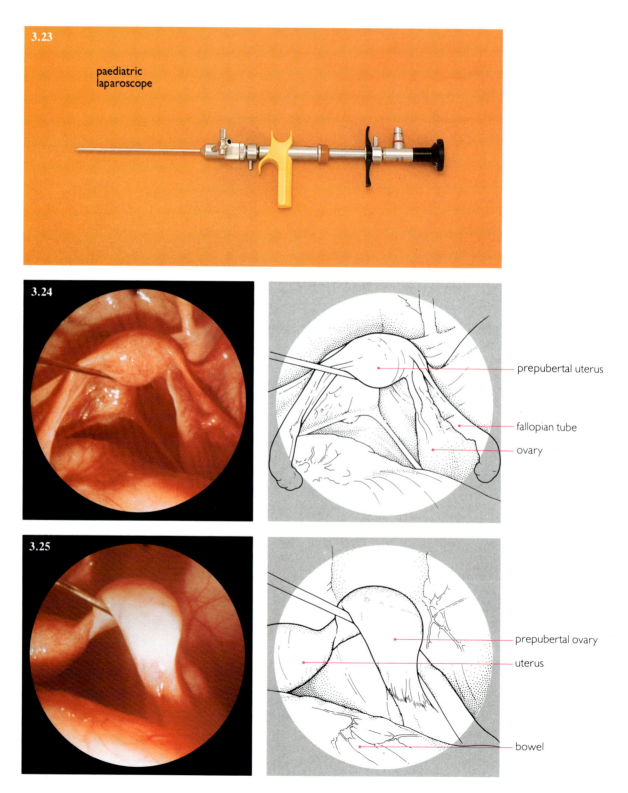

3.23

paediatric laparoscope

3.24

prepubertal uterus

fallopian tube

ovary

3.25

prepubertal ovary

uterus

bowel

Complications

Laparoscopy is a potentially dangerous operation and major complications can only be avoided by meticulous attention to detail. Doctors in training must be carefully supervised by an experienced laparoscopist. The British laparoscopy survey in 1978 showed that, in those regions where a large number of laparoscopies were performed, the complication rate was 3.2%, compared to 5% in regions where laparoscopy was less common. Of the 50,247 laparoscopies reviewed, there were 29.9/1000 complications in diagnostic procedures and 40.6/1000 in sterilization.

Some of the most serious complications arise due to anaesthesia (Fig.3.26),either during induction and intubation, or from metabolic disturbances due to absorption of carbon dioxide leading to cardiac arrhythmias. Inadequate oxygenation may result either from overdistension of the abdomen with gas, making ventilation difficult, or from a steep Trendelenburg position in an obese patient. Normally, 1–2 litres of gas is adequate, but in the obese patient, or in those undergoing operative laparoscopy, more may be required. Once an adequate amount of gas has been insufflated, the source should be turned off or switched to automatic, which compensates for leakage without overdistension. The heart rate should always be monitored during the operation.

Haemorrhage can occur from both superficial and deep vessels. Bleeding from the umbilical incision rarely causes major problems, but may produce an extensive bruise from extravasation of blood into the superficial tissues (Fig.3.27). This always resolves in a few days.

More serious arterial bleeding occurs if the inferior epigastric artery is damaged. The abdominal wall must be transilluminated with the laparoscope to locate the artery before the lateral insertion but, in an obese patient, even this manoevre may not prevent vessel damage. The bleeding may be apparent from the incision, or may be seen through the laparoscope dripping into the pelvis. It is controlled by a deep suture with a semicircular needle, taking in the full thickness of the abdominal wall under laparoscopic control. Occasionally, the incision must be extended and the artery ligated under direct vision.

Major haemorrhage requiring laparotomy and resuscitation occurs when the aorta or the iliac vessels are punctured by the Verres needle or trocar. Such catastrophes can always be avoided by lifting the abdominal wall and inserting the instruments only deep enough to penetrate it and, at the same time, angling the point away from the major vessels.

Perforation of a viscus is a potential hazard and is more likely when there has been previous abdominal surgery or adhesion formation. It is a constant danger during second-look laparoscopy following cancer surgery or irradiation.

Perforation of the small bowel with a Verres needle may pass unnoticed, and is usually harmless. It can be avoided by the aspiration test. Penetration of the bowel or stomach

3.26 Complications following general anaesthesia

Bronchospasm, urticaria, hypotension following thiopentone induction
Vasodilation following althesin
Failure to intubate
Regurgitation of stomach contents
Gaseous distension of stomach
Tachycardia
Suxamethonium apnoea
Incomplete reversal of non-depolarizing relaxants
Intraoperative and postoperative hypotension
Hyperventilation causing tetany
Laryngospasm at extubation
Postoperative vomiting
Opiate overdose

(Fig.3.28) by the trocar requires laparotomy and suture of the perforation. It may be suspected if the patient passes flatus during the operation or, if the stomach has been perforated, gas escapes from the oesophagus. A faecal smell from gas escaping from the needle or cannula is also diagnostic.

Perforation of the uterus by the uterine sound (Fig.3.29) or fine dilator is not uncommon and is more likely in the postmenopausal woman or if the uterus is retroverted.

Uterine perforation with a coil occurs especially in the puerperal uterus. In Fig.3.30 a Gravigard has penetrated the myometrium and is

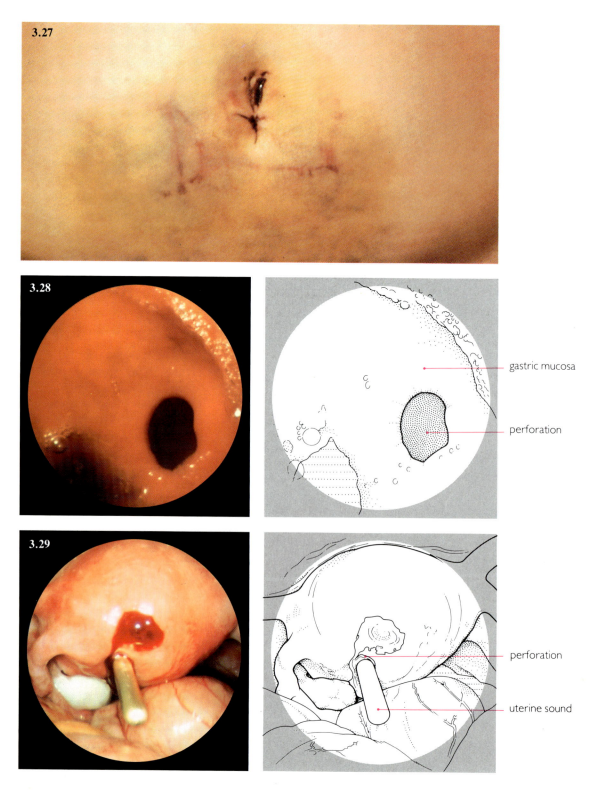

3.27

3.28

gastric mucosa

perforation

3.29

perforation

uterine sound

protruding from the uterus. The coil is grasped with forceps and pulled through the uterine wall before being removed from the abdomen through a cannula (Fig.3.31). Occasionally, the uterine perforation bleeds but this usually stops spontaneously. Persistent oozing is controlled by endocoagulation with a point coagu-lator (Fig.3.32). If the coil is embedded in the omentum it may be removed by traction (Figs.3.33 & 3.34) preceded, if necessary, by scissor dissection and control of bleeding by coagulation. If it is deeply embedded, however, laparotomy may be necessary.

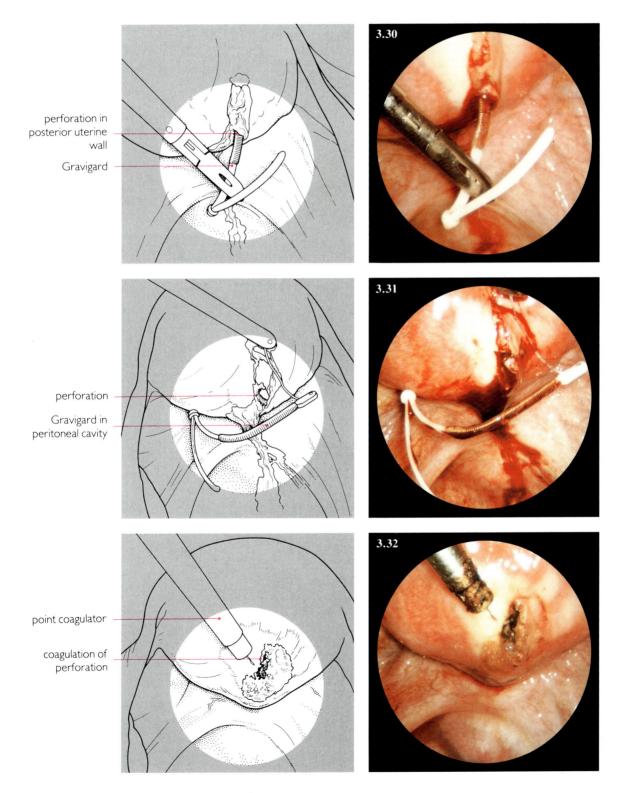

perforation in posterior uterine wall

Gravigard

3.30

perforation

Gravigard in peritoneal cavity

3.31

point coagulator

coagulation of perforation

3.32

One of the more common complications is extravasation of gas into the extraperitoneal space when the Verres needle is inserted incorrectly (Fig.3.35). The needle should be removed and reinserted or, alternatively, the abdominal wall can be elevated and a trocar and cannula carefully inserted, inspecting its position through the laparoscope until the peritoneum is seen. Other alternatives are to insert the needle suprapubically, where there is less fat, or through the posterior vaginal fornix.

Electrical burns to the bowel are a constant danger and have been a major influence in the replacement of tubal diathermy with rings and clips in female sterilization. Unipolar diathermy is particularly dangerous because of the intense local heat generated and the spread of the electrical current along tissue planes outside the visual field of the operator. Bipolar diathermy or endocoagulation are safer.

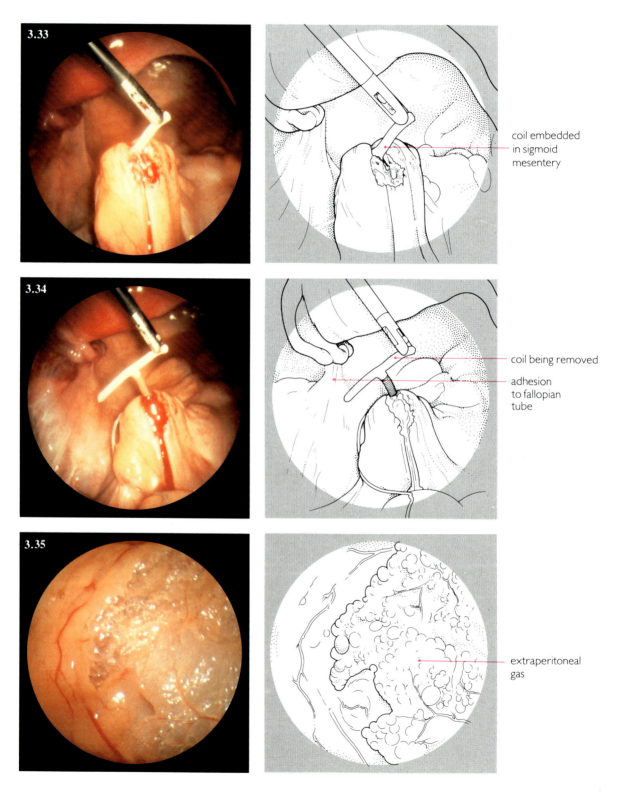

3.33 coil embedded in sigmoid mesentery

3.34 coil being removed / adhesion to fallopian tube

3.35 extraperitoneal gas

Two rare, but serious, complications of laparoscopy are gas embolus and intra-abdominal burns or explosion, caused by escape of methane gas from a bowel perforation followed by the use of electricity. Carbon dioxide is safer for insufflation than nitrous oxide because it does not support combustion. It is essential to insufflate gas slowly at first and to ensure, using the aspiration test, that the tip of the Verres needle lies free within the peritoneum.

The incidence of laparoscopic complications is as listed in Fig.3.36

Reference
Chamberlain GVP & Carron Brown J (1978) *Gynaecological Laparoscopy*. London: Royal College of Obstetricians and Gynaecologists.

3.36

Complications of laparoscopy (RCOG confidential enquiry, 1978)		Rate per 1000 laparoscopies
Anaesthetic complications	Anaesthetic	0.8
	Cardiac arrhythmias	0.4
	Cardiac arrest	0.2
Failed procedures	Failed laparoscopy	7.5
	Failed abdominal insufflation	3.5
	Failed vaginal insufflation	0.0
Burns	Skin	0.3
	Other	0.2
Direct trauma	Pelvic organs	3.4
	Bowel	1.8
	Urinary tract	0.2
Haemorrhage	Pelvic blood vessels and mesosalpinx	2.7
	Abdominal wall	2.5
	Mesentery of bowel	1.1
	Pelvic side-wall and ovarian vessels	0.9
Infection	Abdominal wound	0.5
	Pelvic	0.5
	Urinary tract	0.5
	Chest	0.2
Other complications	Chest pain	0.3
	Pulmonary embolism	0.2
	Deep vein thrombosis	0.2
	Late complications	0.1

INFERTILITY

Introduction

Laparoscopy has replaced gas insufflation in assessing tubal patency and has the additional advantage of allowing a direct view of the pelvic organs. Hysterosalpingography provides information about the proximal tube, but is inaccurate in assessing the distal tube and ovaries.

Laparoscopy and hydropertubation should normally be performed in the first half of the menstrual cycle to avoid the possibility of disturbing a pregnancy. A double puncture technique allows manipulation of the tube and ovary. First, the tube is examined in panoramic view, and then in more detail along its entire length from cornu to fimbriae. Dilute methylene blue is injected; free flow of dye into the peritoneal cavity is usually preceded by air bubbles (Fig.4.1). The dye distends the tubes and drips from the fimbriae to collect in the pouch of Douglas (Figs.4.2 & 4.3).

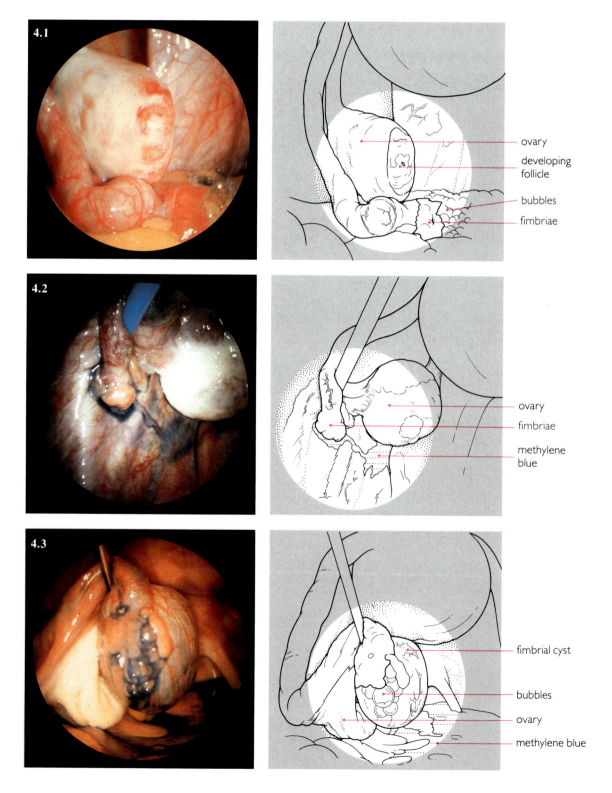

Examination of the ovary provides a guide to ovarian function, and the appearance should therefore be correlated with the phase of the menstrual cycle. The ovary is white and atrophic in non-ovulatory patients and after the menopause. In the pre-ovulatory phase, the dominant follicle may be 25mm in diameter and its vascularity becomes very obvious immediately prior to rupture and ovulation (Fig.4.4).

If laparoscopy is performed just after ovulation (Fig.4.5), the stigma is seen marking the site of escape of the ovum and a few days later the yellowish colour of the corpus luteum is obvious. Two stigmata (Fig.4.6) indicate multiple ovulation.

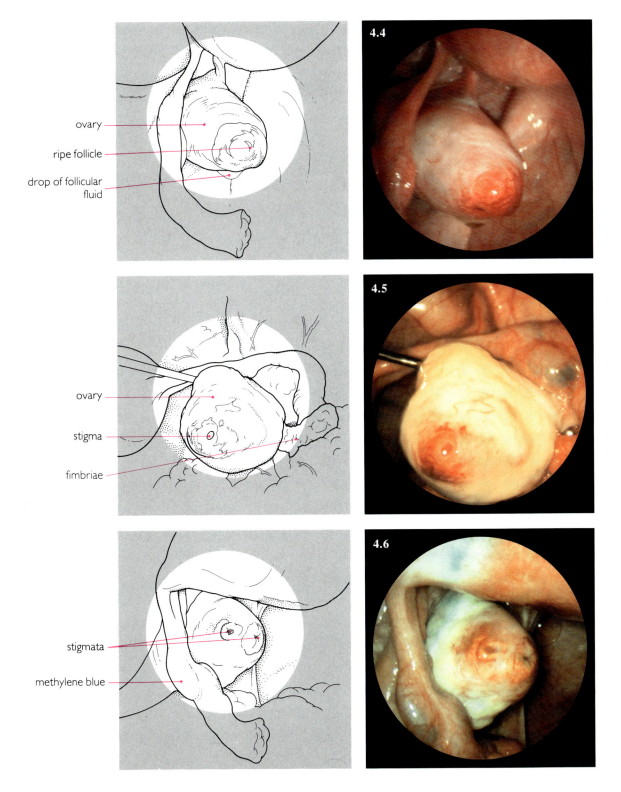

Infection

Recurrent episodes of acute salpingitis often precede permanent tubal damage. Pus from the peritoneal cavity should be cultured, although it is uncommon to identify the organisms. *Neisseria gonorrhoeae* is probably the most common cause, but *Chlamydia* may be involved.

The appearance of salpingitis is unmistakable (Fig.4.7). The tube is red, haemorrhagic and oedematous. The surrounding structures, including the uterus and the peritoneal surface of the bowel, also show an acute inflammatory reaction with a fibrinous exudate (Fig.4.8) and dissection with a probe may be needed to separate the tube and ovary from bowel. Frank pus may be seen leaking from the tubal ostium (Fig.4.9) and manipulation will lead to a sudden gush of pus into the peritoneum from a tubo-ovarian abscess.

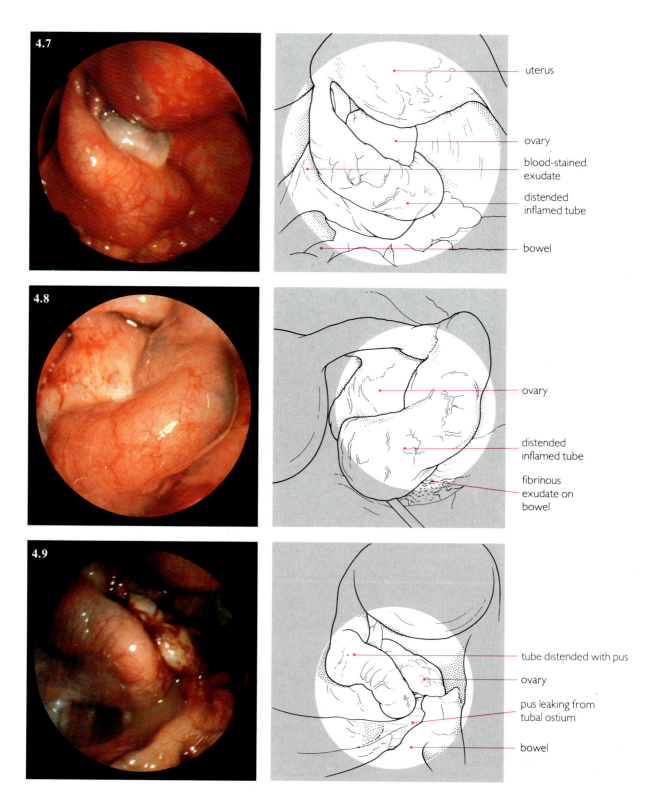

4.7
uterus
ovary
blood-stained exudate
distended inflamed tube
bowel

4.8
ovary
distended inflamed tube
fibrinous exudate on bowel

4.9
tube distended with pus
ovary
pus leaking from tubal ostium
bowel

High-dose broad-spectrum antibiotic therapy and metronidazole is essential if full resolution is to occur.

Inadequately treated salpingitis leads to subfertility due to peritubal or periovarian adhesions. Infertility can also result from ascending infection in the puerperium or following septic abortion. Typically, the adhesions are very fine and often involve both the tube and ovary (Fig.4.10). In many patients the fimbriae cannot be seen without first performing adhesiolysis.

Even with extensive adhesions, the tubal ostium may be patent and thus methylene blue spills into the peritoneal cavity although it is loculated (Fig.4.11). The ovary is often buried in fine transparent sheets of peritoneum, even though the tube is patent, which may result in misdiagnosis if hysterosalpingography is used to assess patency (Fig.4.12). These fine

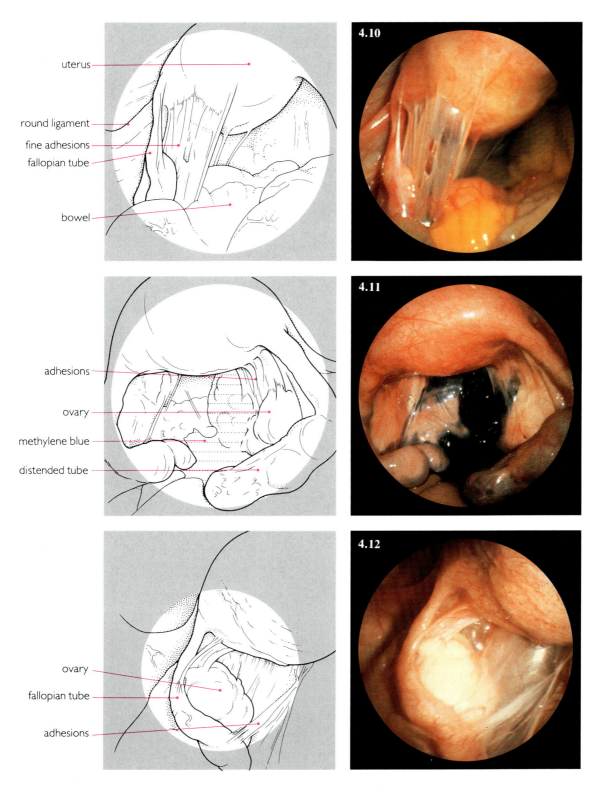

adhesions are easily divided with hook scissors, resulting in restoration of fertility. Dense omental adhesions limit access to the pelvis and may entirely cover the adnexa (Fig.4.13). Operations on the uterus, tubes and ovaries, especially Caesarean section, ovarian cystectomy and myomectomy, are a frequent cause. Surgical techniques and haemostasis must be meticulous.

Large myomata, especially submucous fibroids, may cause infertility by distorting the uterus. Fibroids may be accompanied by endometriosis or pelvic inflammatory disease, both of which also cause fibrosis and adhesions (Fig.4.14). Rupture of an endometriotic cyst releases concentrated blood into the peritoneum and results in both the tube and ovary being covered by omentum (Fig.4.15).

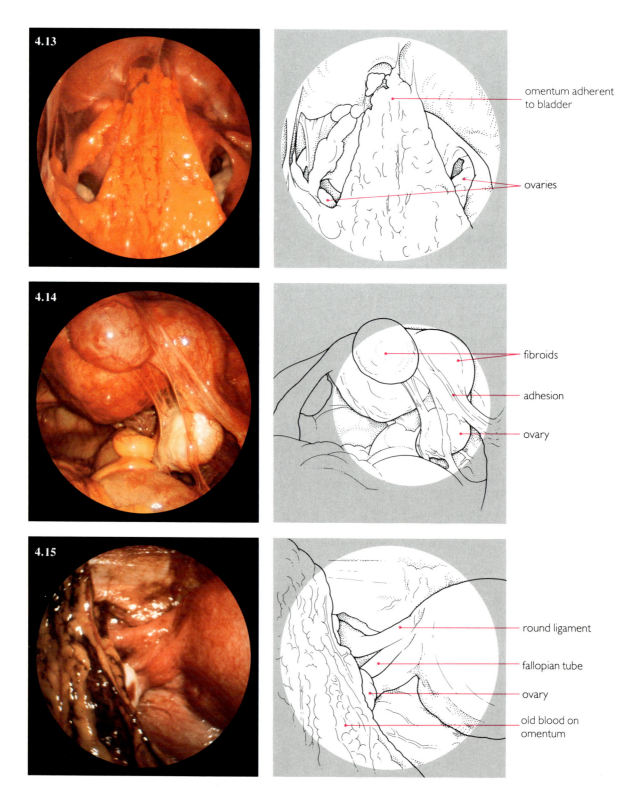

4.13 — omentum adherent to bladder / ovaries

4.14 — fibroids / adhesion / ovary

4.15 — round ligament / fallopian tube / ovary / old blood on omentum

Ventrosuspension is occasionally performed to correct a retroverted uterus without other pathology, but is more often combined with myomectomy or ovarian cystectomy. The tube may be pulled forwards with the round ligament and the resulting distortion (Fig.4.16) can cause infertility.

Acute appendicitis may lead to pelvic sepsis and tubal blockage. Occasionally the appendix adheres to the tube (Fig.4.17), but whether the primary pathology lies in the appendix or the tube is often doubtful. Any abdominal operation can cause omental adhesions (Fig.4.18), which limit access to the pelvis

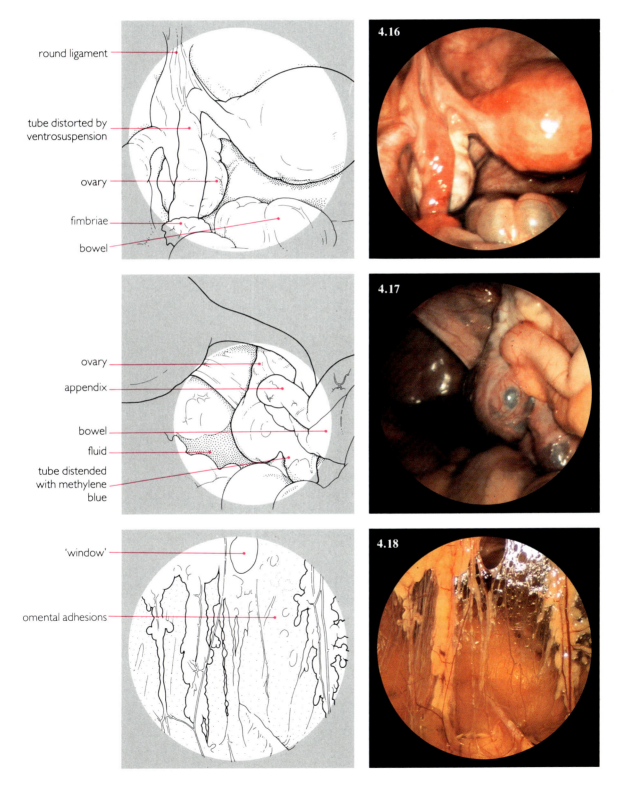

round ligament

tube distorted by
ventrosuspension

ovary

fimbriae

bowel

4.16

ovary

appendix

bowel

fluid

tube distended
with methylene
blue

4.17

'window'

omental adhesions

4.18

unless there is an avascular 'widow' through which to insert the telescope.

Chlamydial salpingitis (Fig.4.19) is becoming increasingly common. The tube is thickened and oedematous but, unlike acute gonococcal salpingitis, free pus is rarely seen. Culture of the organism is difficult and specialized laboratory facilities are required. Chlamydial salpingitis is often associated with

extensive adhesion formation between the superior surface of the liver and the diaphragm (Fig.4.20). Therefore the upper abdomen should always be examined if chlamydial infection is suspected.

Of all the infections which can give rise to salpingitis and infertility, pelvic tuberculosis is now the least common in western European

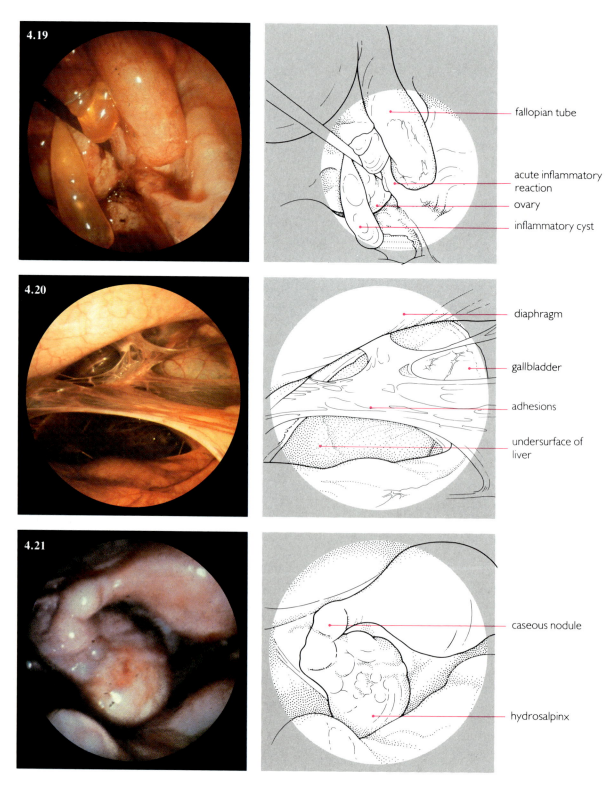

4.19
- fallopian tube
- acute inflammatory reaction
- ovary
- inflammatory cyst

4.20
- diaphragm
- gallbladder
- adhesions
- undersurface of liver

4.21
- caseous nodule
- hydrosalpinx

countries, although it is still common in developing countries. A tuberculous hydrosalpinx can be distinguished by the caseous nodules along the fallopian tube (Fig.4.21) and is always bilateral.

The diagnosis should be confirmed by histology and bacteriological culture of the endometrium. It is usually unwise to attempt biopsy of the suspected tubercular nodules because of the risk of spreading active tuberculosis throughout the abdomen (Fig.4.22).

Tubal obstruction

Tubal blockage may be either cornual or fimbrial. Hydrosalpinx may be unilateral or bilateral and can vary in size from a minor dilatation of the ampulla to gross distension of the whole length of the tube (Fig.4.23). The cornual orifice is always open and this allows the tube to fill with radio-opaque dye at hysterosalpingography or with methylene blue at laparoscopy (Fig.4.24). Even without dye,

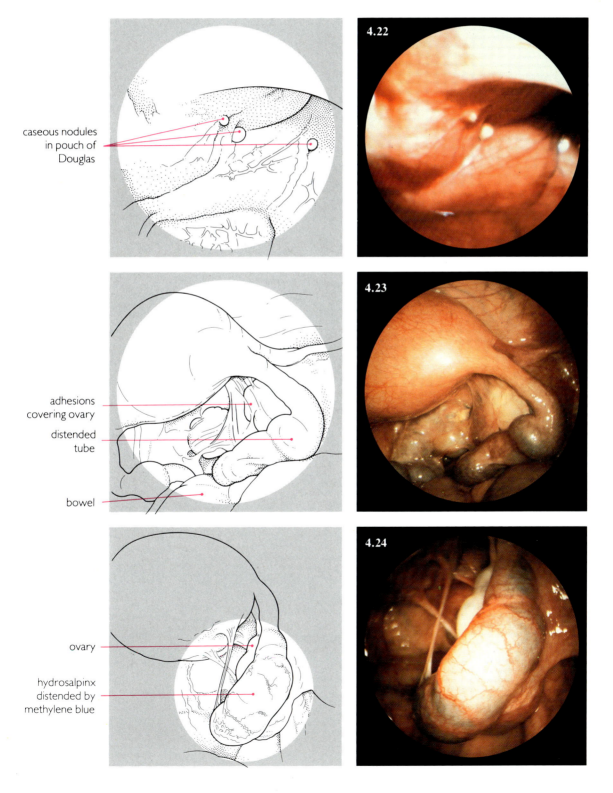

caseous nodules in pouch of Douglas

4.22

adhesions covering ovary

distended tube

bowel

4.23

ovary

hydrosalpinx distended by methylene blue

4.24

the thin-walled distended tube appears blue because of the fluid and altered blood in its lumen. This appearance becomes more obvious as the hydrosalpinx grows larger and the wall of the tube becomes thinner (Fig.4.25), but in spite of the increasing tension, a hydrosalpinx rarely ruptures.

Cornual obstruction is more difficult to diagnose because stenosis must be distinguished from a physiological block caused by tubal spasm. A hysterosalpingogram might suggest cornual block but laparoscopy gives a more accurate diagnosis. Dye injected through the cervix fills the uterus but does not enter the tube even under pressure (Fig.4.26). The dye enters myometrial capillaries and the uterus turns blue (Fig.4.27).

By advancing the telescope into the pelvis and closer to the tube, it is sometimes possible to see the precise site of the occlusion and to view the extravasation in more detail (Fig.4.28). Cornual block is treated by

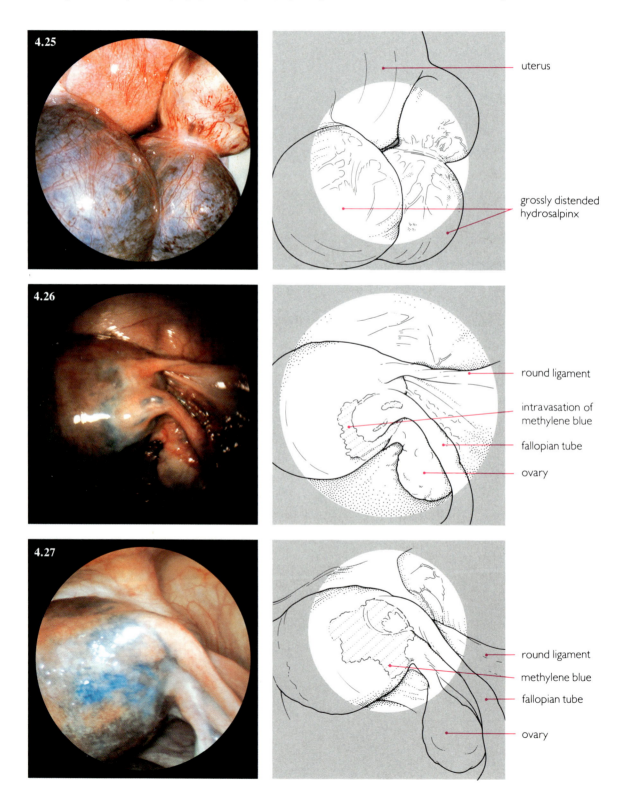

laparotomy and tubal microsurgery or cornual implantation.

Surgery for hydrosalpinx should be considered only when there is a reasonable possibility of success. In extreme cases the cilia and tubal epithelium atrophy due to progressive pressure and the tube will not function even if it can be opened successfully. Surgery for hydrosalpinx is conventionally performed by laparotomy, but an expert endoscopist can operate with the laparoscope using two or more portals to introduce the operating instruments.

The tip of the tube is incised with sharp scissors (Fig.4.29) and the distending fluid and methylene blue are released into the peritoneal cavity (Fig.4.30). The fimbriae can then be sutured onto the peritoneum of the tube to form a cuff salpingostomy. Sometimes,

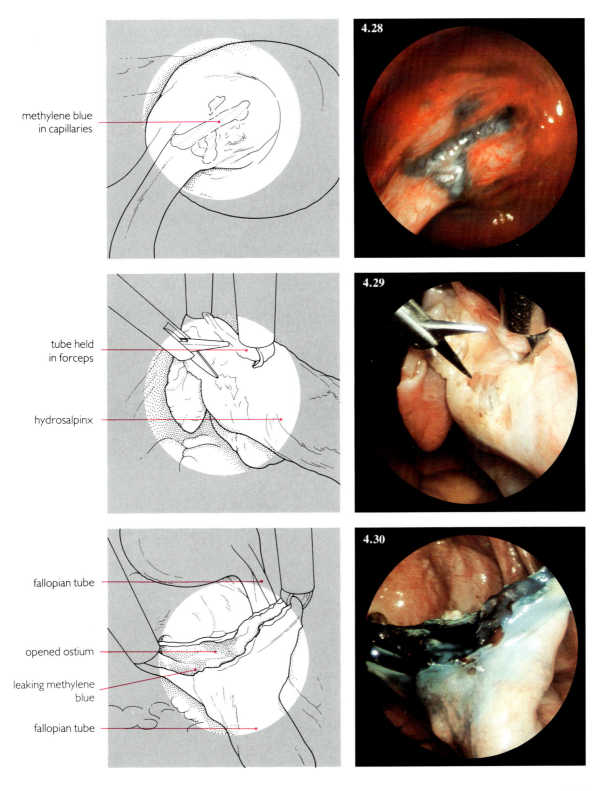

methylene blue in capillaries

4.28

tube held in forceps

hydrosalpinx

4.29

fallopian tube

opened ostium

leaking methylene blue

fallopian tube

4.30

however, sutures are not needed and the tube heals spontaneously (Fig.4.31).

Salpingostomy is more usually performed by laparotomy and microsurgery. The final result of the operation, if performed with fine instruments, magnification and careful attention to haemostasis, will result in a normal-looking tubal ostium (Fig.4.32), but there is an increased risk of ectopic pregnancy.

There are many postoperative regimes employed to avoid development of further adhesions. These include antibiotics, systemic

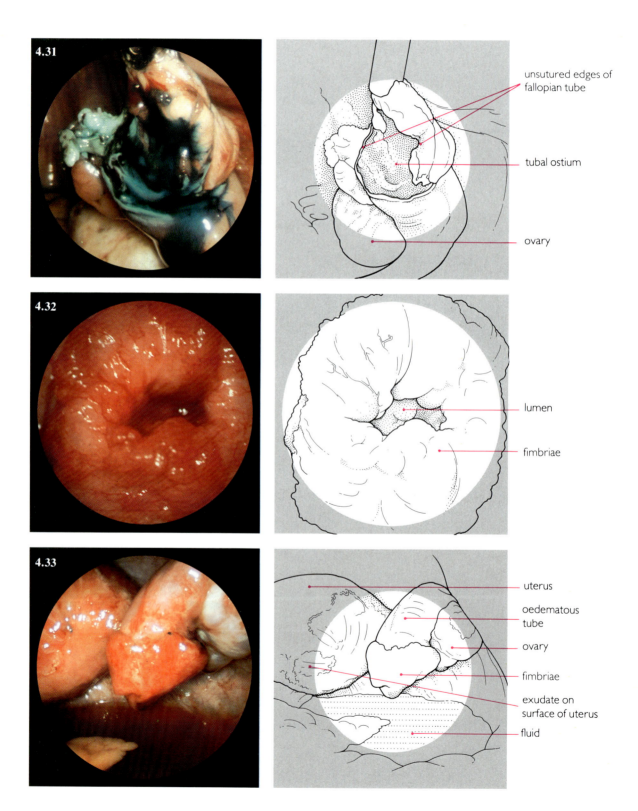

or local steroid therapy, intraperitoneal dextran and transcervical hydropertubation. It is uncommon for surgeons to laparoscope their patients in the postoperative phase, but early laparoscopy reveals tissue reaction with oedema and an inflammatory exudate (Fig.4.33). Hydropertubation or peritoneal lavage (Fig.4.34) with a steroid solution may be of value in maintaining tubal patency and preventing adhesion formation.

Ovarian Disorders

The combination of obesity, hirsutism and oligomenorrhoea in association with anovulation suggests the diagnosis of polycystic ovarian syndrome. Characteristically, both ovaries are enlarged with a white surface and no follicular development (Figs.4.35 & 4.36). The white appearance distinguishes the ovaries from simple follicular or luteal cysts, but the most important differential diagnosis is from a

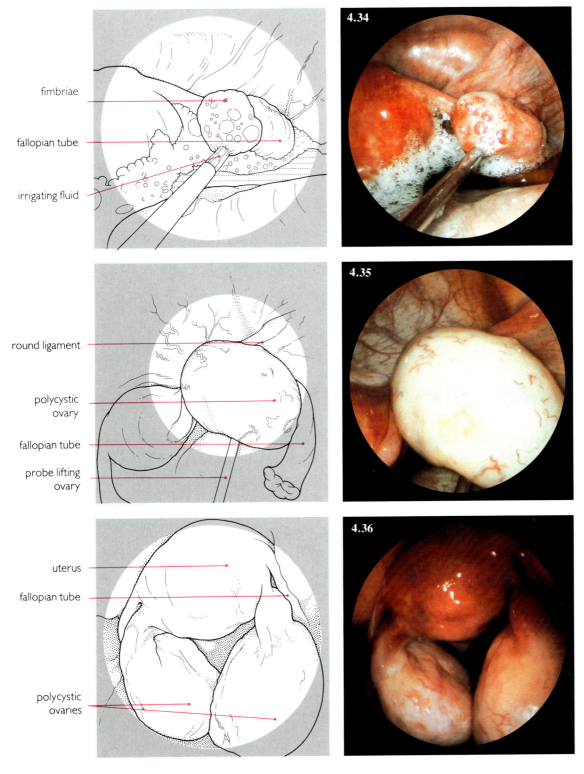

dermoid. Dermoids never cause menstrual disturbance, although they are frequently bilateral. The androgen levels and the LH:FSH ratio in the blood are usually elevated in polycystic ovarian disease but the diagnosis can be established by biopsy (Fig.4.37), which shows a thickened tunica albuginea without follicular development.

In polycystic ovarian disease, spontaneous ovulation often occurs following wedge resection, or it may be induced with clomiphene or FSH. Hyperstimulation of the ovary is rare with clomiphene, but more common with human menopausal gonadotrophin or FSH (Fig.4.38). The tender, enlarged ovary always undergoes spontaneous resolution and surgery is needed only for haemorrhage or torsion.

In anorexia nervosa with gross loss of weight and amenorrhoea, laparoscopy shows smooth ovaries (Fig.4.39) with no follicular development.

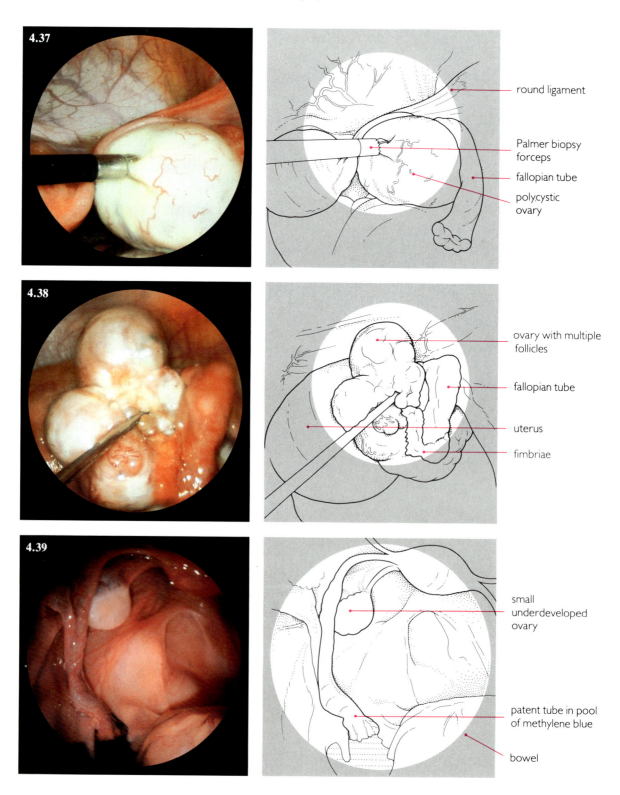

Congenital Abnormalities

Congenital abnormalities of the uterus due to failure of fusion of the Müllerian ducts should be suspected if there has been recurrent abortion. Alternatively, it can be an incidental finding in the investigation of infertility. Any degree of failure of fusion can be found, varying from complete reduplication to a minor abnormality such as an arcuate uterus.

In uterus bicornis bicollis (Fig.4.40) the two horns have a band of tissue running between them from bladder to rectum, but in a lesser degree of reduplication this is absent (Fig.4.41). The bicornuate uterus with a single cervix and the subseptate uterus (Fig.4.42) have a depression at the fundus, but the extent of the failure of fusion can only be diagnosed by hysterosalpingography or hysteroscopy.

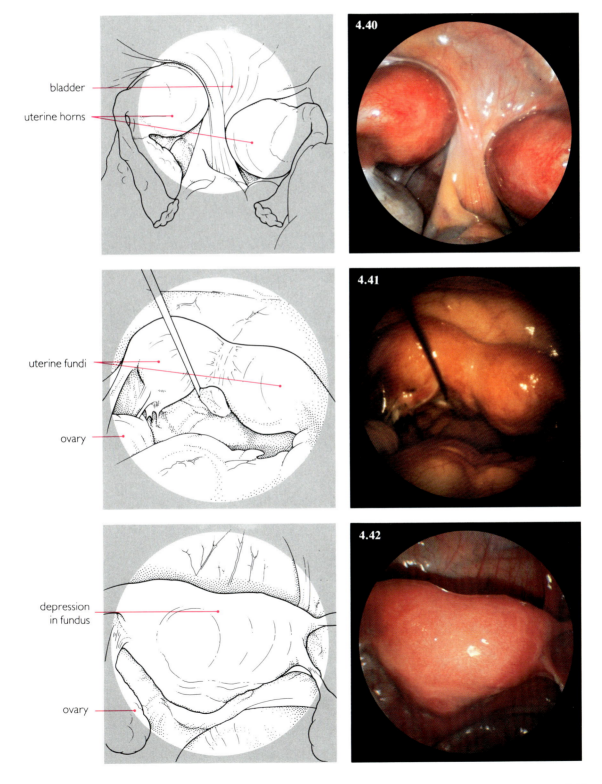

A unicornuate uterus has a single horn with the round ligament, tube and ovarian ligament in their correct anatomical relationship at the cornu (Fig.4.43). A rudimentary horn on the contralateral side (Fig.4.44) is an occasional finding.

Pregnancy in a rudimentary horn (Fig.4.45) is rare and, before the advent of ultrasound, was difficult to diagnose. The pregnancy can continue to grow until the third trimester but uterine rupture and catastrophic haemorrhage inevitably occur. There is always associated oligohydramnios and placenta accreta.

In all such uterine abnormalities the possibility of a coexisting renal anomaly must be remembered and radiological studies should

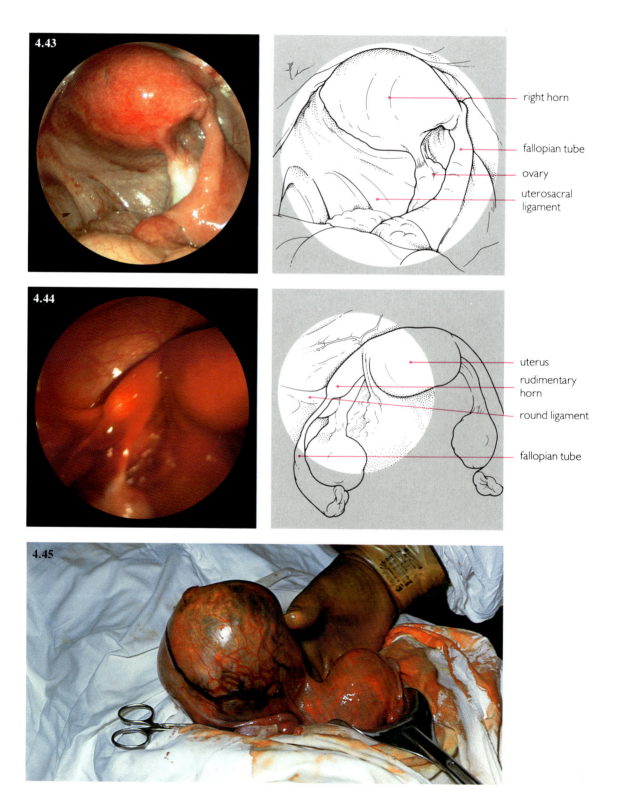

4.43 — right horn, fallopian tube, ovary, uterosacral ligament

4.44 — uterus, rudimentary horn, round ligament, fallopian tube

4.45

be performed. Unilateral absence of the kidney is a common accompaniment: more rarely, a pelvic kidney may be found (Fig.4.46).

Complete absence of the uterus, the Rokitanski–Kuster–Hauser syndrome (Fig. 4.47), is uncommon. In this syndrome, the external genitalia and the length of the vagina are normal, but there is no cervix palpable on vaginal examination. At laparoscopy, there may be a nodule of tissue representing the uterus and the typical cruciate formation of the round and uterosacral ligaments. Normal adnexa may be present, even in complete absence of the uterus (Fig.4.48).

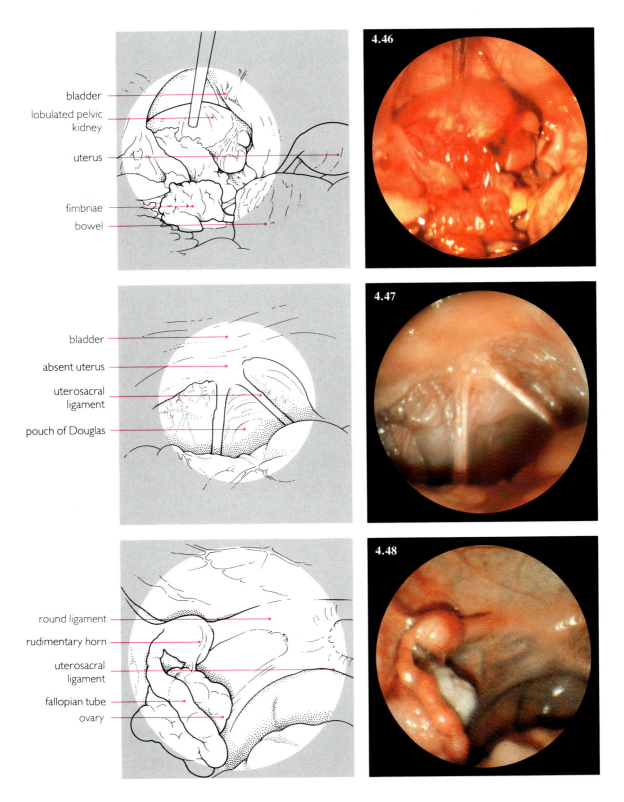

bladder
lobulated pelvic kidney
uterus
fimbriae
bowel

4.46

bladder
absent uterus
uterosacral ligament
pouch of Douglas

4.47

round ligament
rudimentary horn
uterosacral ligament
fallopian tube
ovary

4.48

In uterine hypoplasia, laparoscopy confirms the infantile uterus but the ovary appears normal (Fig.4.49). There are no follicles apparent in this ovary and therefore measurement of pituitary gonadotrophin is necessary to distinguish between pituitary and ovarian failure.

Streak ovaries will be suggested by primary amenorrhoea, low oestrogen and high FSH levels, and failure of ultrasound to show ovarian tissue. Chromosome analysis may show an abnormal karyotype. At laparoscopy (Figs.4.50 & 4.51) the amount of ovarian tissue varies in size from an area of white thickening in the ovarian ligament to a small but recognizable ovary. These patients do not ovulate when given gonadotrophin therapy, whereas the patient with a congenitally small

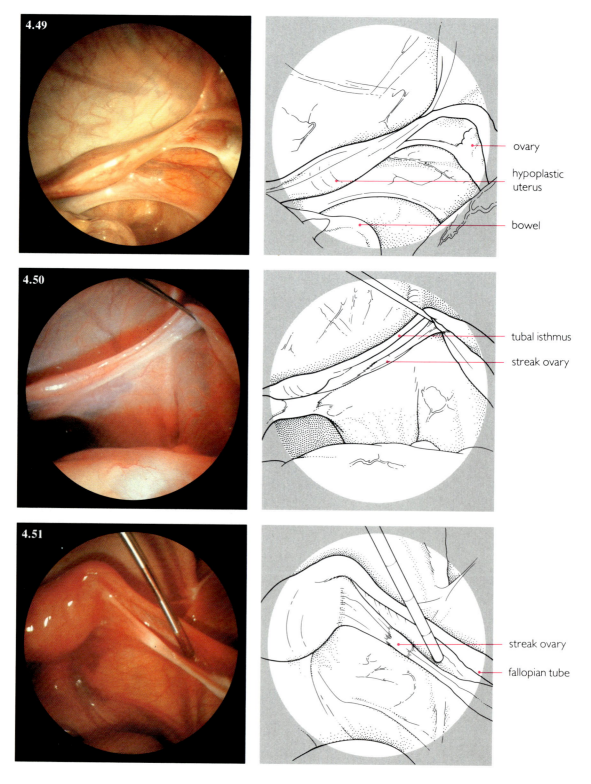

ovary (Fig.4.52) and normal chromosomes does respond to stimulation. The patient with Turner's syndrome has no ovaries, a small uterus, 45 chromosomes and a characteristic physical appearance. Occasionally, however, some uterine development, possibly caused by adrenal oestrogens, does occur in ovarian agenesis (Fig.4.53). In testicular feminization, the phenotype is that of a mature woman with good breast development but minimal axillary and pubic hair. The karyotype is 46XY and laparoscopy usually reveals an abdominal testis, although it may sometimes be situated in the inguinal canal. An ovotestis may sometimes be found in the same situation (Fig.4.54). Both structures should be removed after sexual maturity because of the risk of malignancy.

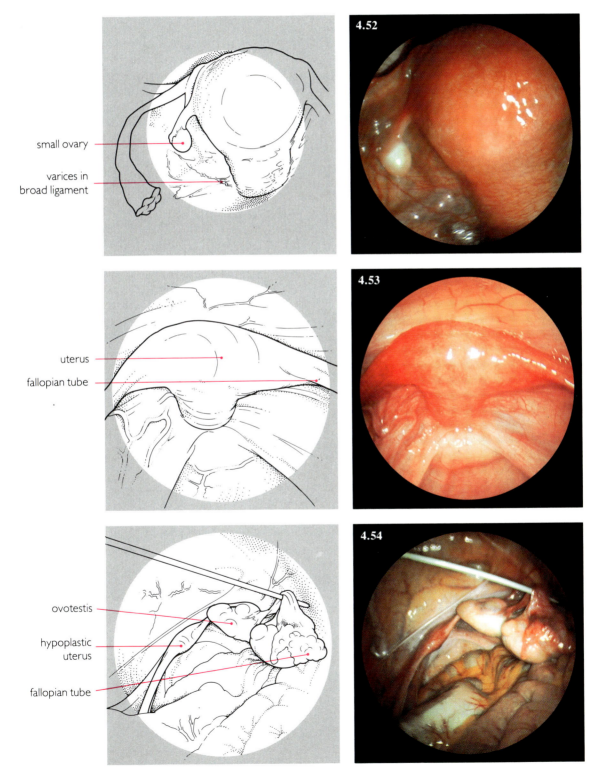

Ectopic pregnancy

A ruptured extrauterine pregnancy with severe abdominal pain, bleeding and collapse is one of the more dramatic gynaecological emergencies and requires immediate resuscitation and surgery. A leaking tubal abortion presents insidiously with irregular vaginal bleeding or amenorrhoea, lower abdominal pain and signs of peritoneal irritation.

Laparoscopy will always reveal blood smeared over the surface of the small bowel and, on advancing the telescope further into the pelvis, a variable amount of blood can be seen in the pouch of Douglas (Figs.4.55 & 4.56). The standard practice on seeing blood in the peritoneal cavity is to proceed without delay to laparotomy and salpingectomy.

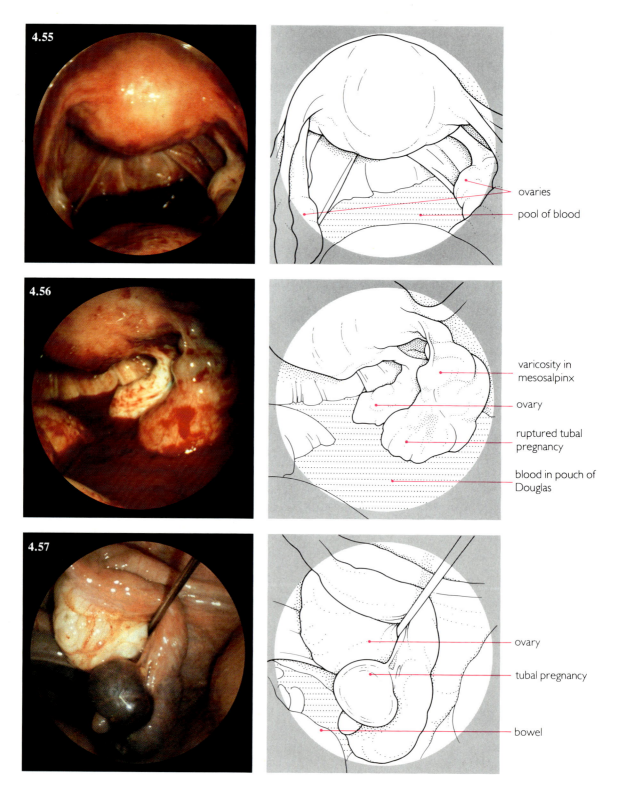

4.55 — ovaries / pool of blood

4.56 — varicosity in mesosalpinx / ovary / ruptured tubal pregnancy / blood in pouch of Douglas

4.57 — ovary / tubal pregnancy / bowel

Ectopic pregnancy is more likely in patients who have previously had tubal surgery or who have chronic pelvic inflammatory disease. It has now also become a significant risk in patients undergoing in vitro fertilization with embryo replacement. Early laparoscopy in patients with pelvic pain allows the diagnosis of an unruptured ectopic (Figs.4.57 & 4.58) to be made at a stage when conservative surgery is possible.

If a slow leak of blood into the peritoneal cavity continues over a period of days or weeks, the omentum adheres to the tube (Fig.4.59), producing a peritubal mass which is palpable and tender. If the pregnancy implants in the ampulla, rupture will eventually occur or, alternatively, the pregnancy will abort into the tubal lumen to be extruded from the fimbrial end (Fig.4.60) with a variable amount of bleeding.

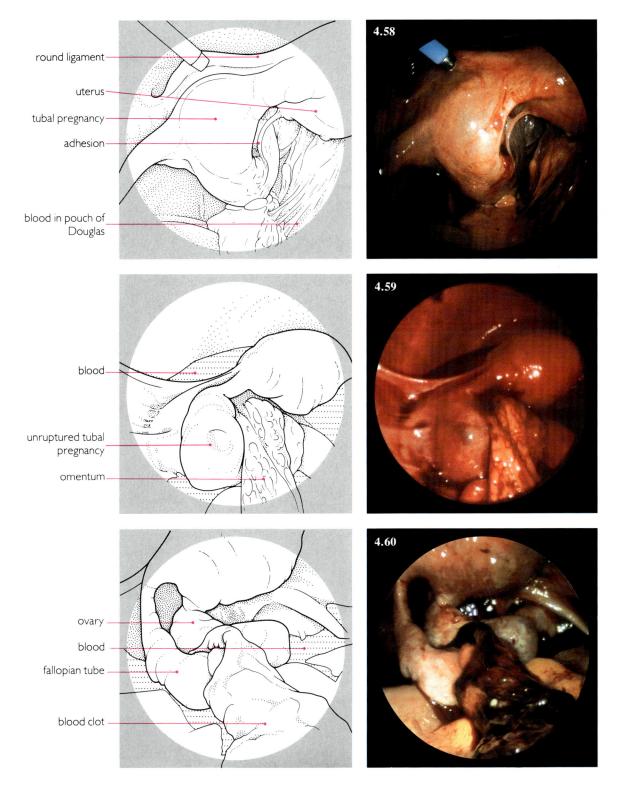

Conservative surgery should now be considered in any patient who wishes to have more children and who has an ectopic pregnancy with an intact tube (Fig.4.61). Most surgeons do this by laparotomy and microsurgery, but if the tubal pregnancy is small, conservative surgery can be performed by laparoscopy. First, the blood is washed out of the pelvis and the tube is held using atraumatic forceps and carefully inspected to determine the site of the pregnancy (Fig.4.62). The tube is then coagulated (Fig.4.63) over the pregnancy sac with a point coagulator.

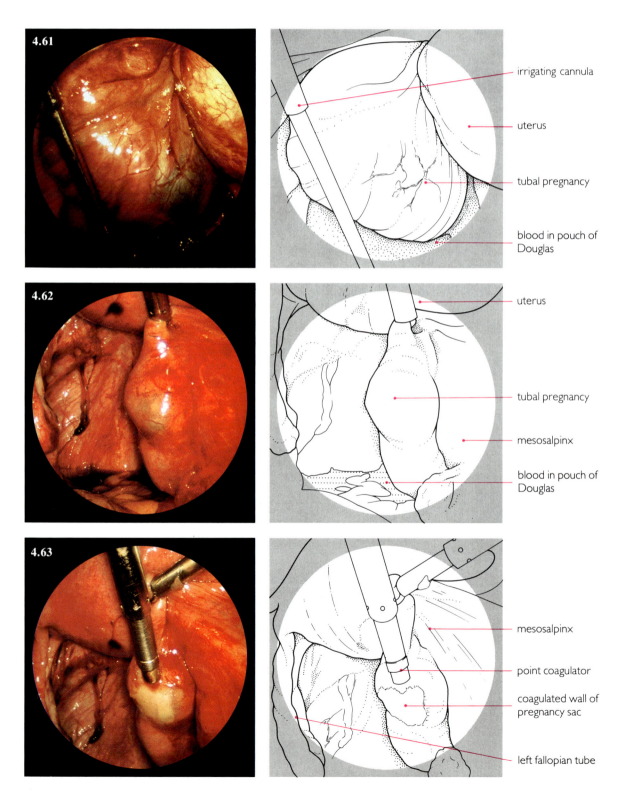

4.61
— irrigating cannula
— uterus
— tubal pregnancy
— blood in pouch of Douglas

4.62
— uterus
— tubal pregnancy
— mesosalpinx
— blood in pouch of Douglas

4.63
— mesosalpinx
— point coagulator
— coagulated wall of pregnancy sac
— left fallopian tube

The coagulated tube is incised with hook scissors (Fig.4.64) while the isthmus is held steady with forceps. The tube contracts and the pregnancy is extruded (Fig.4.65). If the pregnancy does not separate completely from the tube, dissection with forceps will help to peel it off the wall or, alternatively, it can be removed from the tube by suction.

Finally, the incision in the tube is sutured or coagulated. Suturing is preferable because there is less risk of fistula formation. If suturing is not performed, small bleeding points can be ligated with a Roeder loop (Fig.4.66).

If the pregnancy is invading the meso-salpinx, the incision will have to be made into

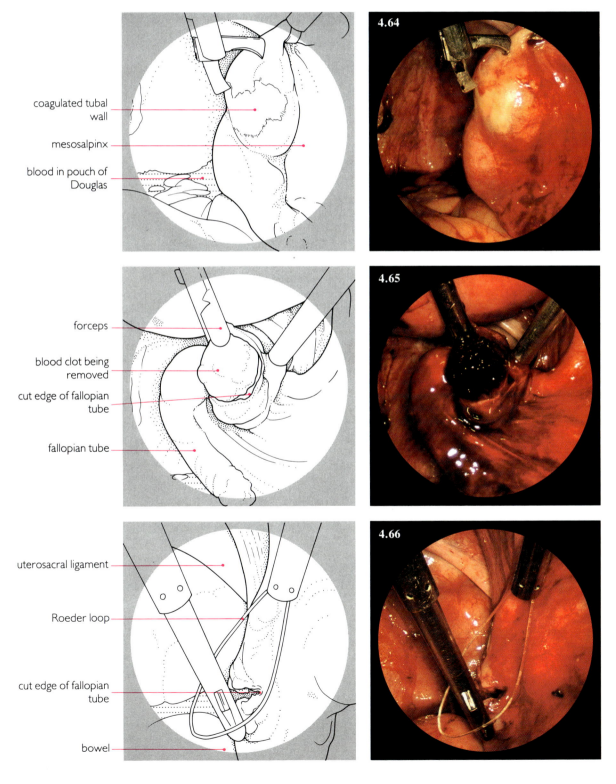

the tubal mesentery (Fig.4.67) and the pregnancy delivered with atraumatic forceps and suction (Fig.4.68). The remaining products of conception are removed and the bleeding edges of the tubal opening are treated, in this case with electrocoagulation (Fig.4.69).

The technique of conservative endoscopic surgery in tubal pregnancy requires considerable technical dexterity and appropriate instruments. Thus, the tube is conserved and the results in terms of future intrauterine pregnancy appear to be at least as good as with laparotomy.

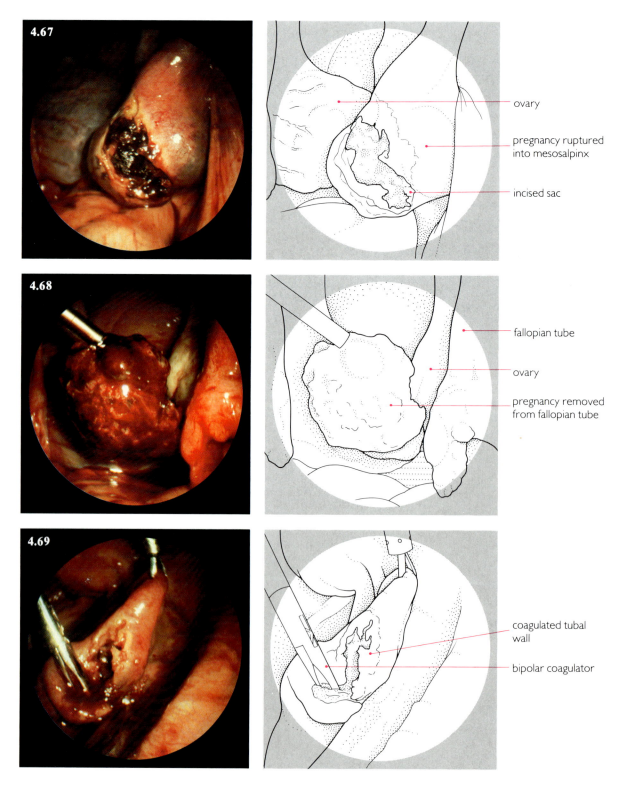

5

PELVIC INFLAMMATORY DISEASE

Acute Infection

Acute salpingitis usually presents with lower abdominal pain, pyrexia and signs of peritonitis. Laparoscopy is frequently necessary to confirm the diagnosis and to exclude other causes of pelvic pain such as ectopic pregnancy and appendicitis.

In acute salpingitis, the tubes are red and oedematous with pus dripping from the fimbriae (Fig.5.1); this can be aspirated for culture. Suitable antibiotic therapy at this stage of the disease allows complete resolution. If treatment is delayed or inadequate, however, the fimbriae will close and the tube becomes filled with pus, forming a pyosalpinx (Fig.5.2) which may be ruptured on laparoscopic exploration with release of pus into the pelvis. In Fig.5.3 the tube is distended and oedematous, and separation of adhesions has caused bleeding and pooling of blood in the pouch of Douglas.

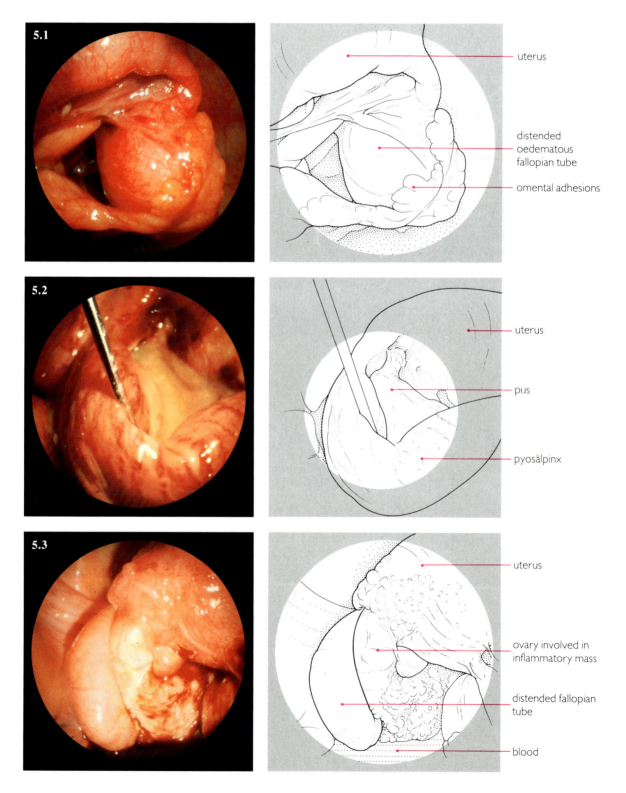

A fibrinous exudate forms on the surface of the bowel and on the tube in response to generalized peritoneal infection (Fig.5.4). Fine adhesions develop between bowel and adnexa, and the omentum may also become involved in the inflammatory process, interfering with access to the pelvis. In Fig.5.5 the omentum is adherent to an abdominal wound and must be divided to improve the view, controlling bleeding vessels by endocoagulation. Alternatively, it is often possible to introduce the telescope through a thin avascular 'window' in the omentum to gain access to the pelvis.

Chronic Pelvic Inflammatory Disease

If the acute infection fails to resolve fully, fibrous adhesions (Fig.5.6) form between the

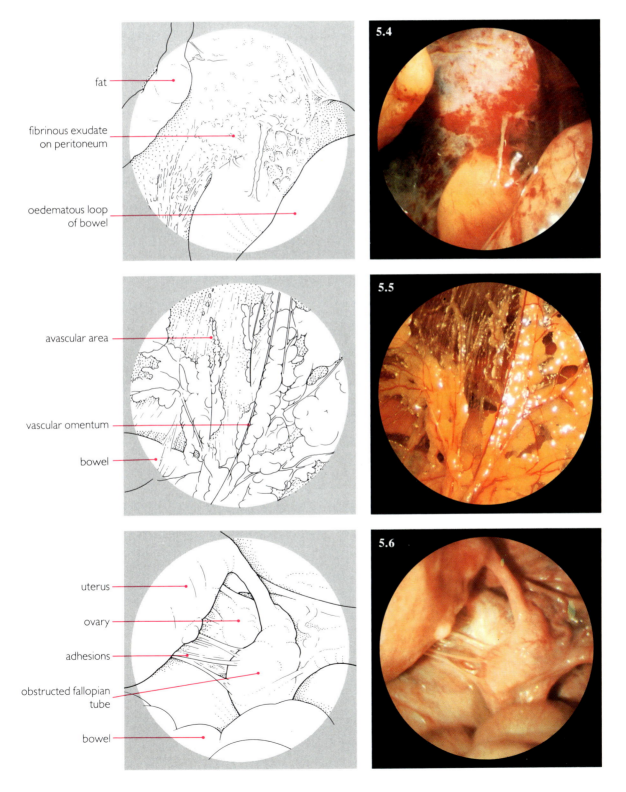

fat

fibrinous exudate on peritoneum

oedematous loop of bowel

avascular area

vascular omentum

bowel

uterus

ovary

adhesions

obstructed fallopian tube

bowel

tube, ovary and posterior surface of the uterus and, if the original infection has been inadequately treated, chronic pelvic inflammatory disease with dense adhesions may follow. The adhesions in Fig.5.7 are kinking the tube and are probably obstructing it. The ovary is buried and is firmly adherent to the broad ligament, so that ovum release is impossible.

Loops of small intestine and sigmoid colon adhere to the uterus and adnexa, obliterating the pouch of Douglas (Fig.5.8). Laparotomy and tubal microsurgery are required to reconstruct the normal anatomy, restore fertility and relieve pain. Pelviscopic surgery avoids laparotomy and gives good results in some of these patients.

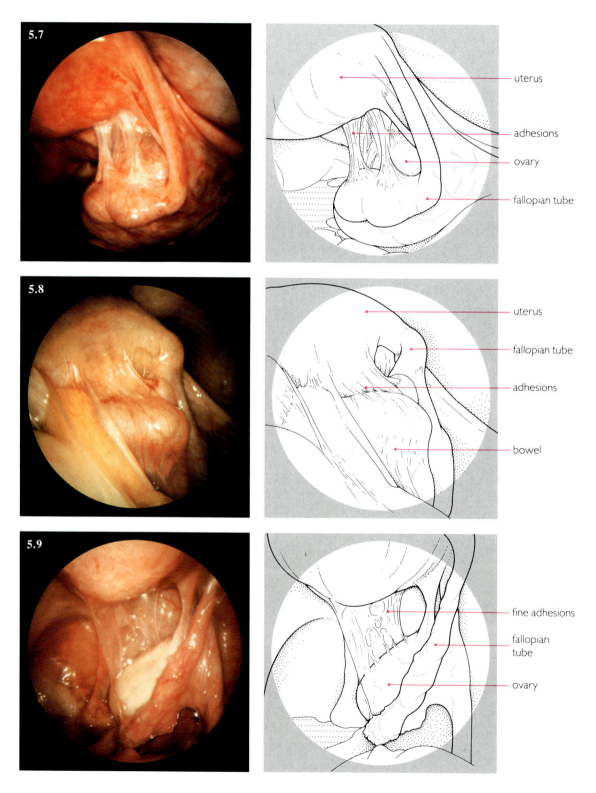

Adhesiolysis

Fine adhesions without tubal obstruction are divided with scissors, freeing and mobilizing the ovary (Figs.5.9 & 5.10). The adhesions which cover the ovary and interfere with ovum release are avascular, and can be removed quite easily by dissection with forceps and scissors. Thicker adhesions, which are also avascular, are displayed in Fig.5.11 using a probe to put them on traction and facilitate division.

More dense adhesions in the pouch of Douglas, between the sigmoid and the posterior surface of the uterus (Fig.5.12), cause chronic pelvic pain and deep dyspareunia. Laparoscopic adhesiolysis is often possible, but laparotomy may be needed because there is a risk of bleeding or damage to the large bowel. In this case, some of the adhesions have been divided and peritoneal lavage performed before proceeding with the operation.

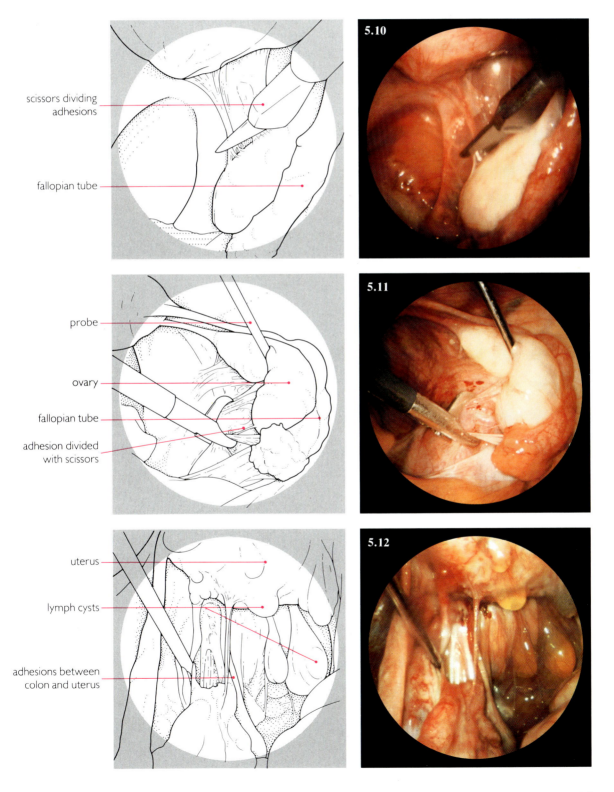

Laser Adhesiolysis

Laser can be used to vaporize adhesions or spots of endometriosis with precision and with very little bleeding. The Argon and Nd.YAG lasers have the advantage of being transmitted along flexible quartz fibres, whereas the carbon dioxide laser requires a special rigid delivery system. All laser surgery must be performed in specially adapted theatres with warning notices for personnel; filters must be inserted into the telescope, or protective goggles worn.

Sutton (1986) initially used a single puncture technique (Fig.5.13), but found that the beam was reflected off the walls of the narrow operating channel, and it was also difficult to prevent the laser beam damaging structures distal to the target tissue. A double puncture technique (Fig.5.14) is preferable as it gives a better view. The use of closed-circuit television enables the surgical team to assist the operator. The laser energy is transmitted via a lens and mirror through a second puncture, positioned so that the beam is at 90° to the target tissue. A third puncture allows tissue traction by an assistant, or irrigation with Hartmann's solution to reduce heat production. If laser is used near the bowel, it is essential to irrigate the tissues with copious amounts of fluid to prevent damage from excessive heat.

Accumulated smoke reduces the power of the laser and interferes with visibility, and should therefore be extracted through the outer sheath of the laser probe.

The laser probe has a non-reflective back stop (Fig.5.15), which prevents the beam from damaging tissues distal to the target. The probe

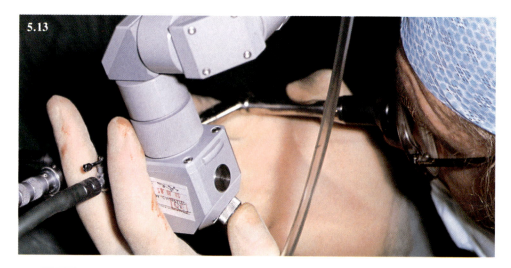

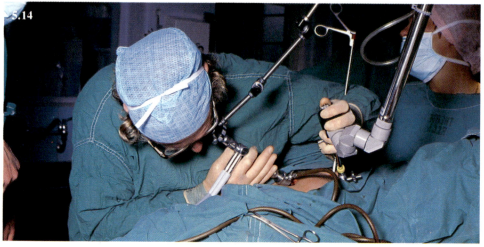

is applied to the adhesion, which is gradually vaporized (Figs.5.16 & 5.17). The advantage of laser vaporization over electrocoagulation is that the tissues are completely destroyed, leaving no residual dead tissue, and making reformation of adhesions less likely.

This is a potentially dangerous technique, but in the hands of an experienced laparoscopist, who is familiar with lasers and their effects on human tissue, it appears to be a useful method, but requires further evaluation.

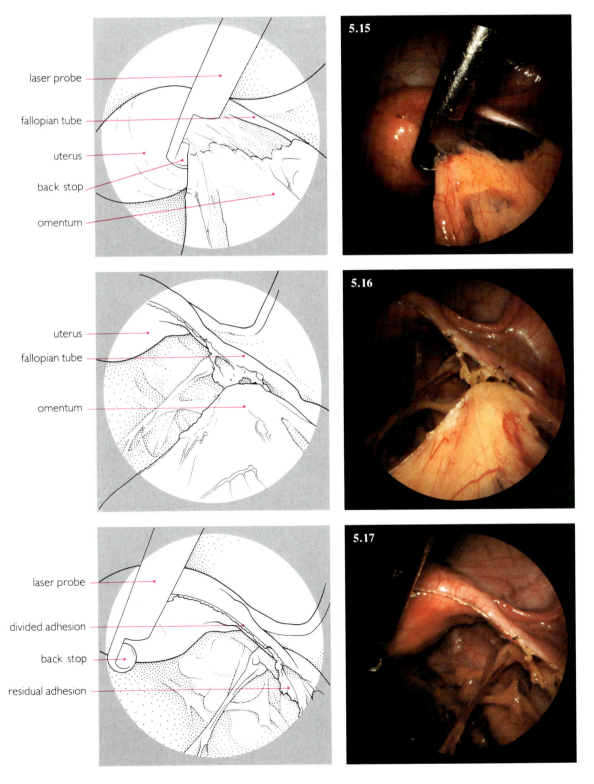

Tubal Obstruction

Chronic pelvic inflammatory disease is often accompanied by distal tubal obstruction and hydrosalpinx. The degree varies from a simple terminal block to a dilated retort-shaped tube. In terminal obstruction, the ampulla is distended and the site of the blocked ostium (Fig.5.18) may be seen as a star-shaped pucker. When salpingostomy is performed, the tube is opened by an incision at this point.

Hydrosalpinx is usually bilateral and the distended tube may be surrounded by adhesions (Fig.5.19). In some patients, the distended tube is patent but locules form around the fimbriae (Fig.5.20) when dye is insufflated.

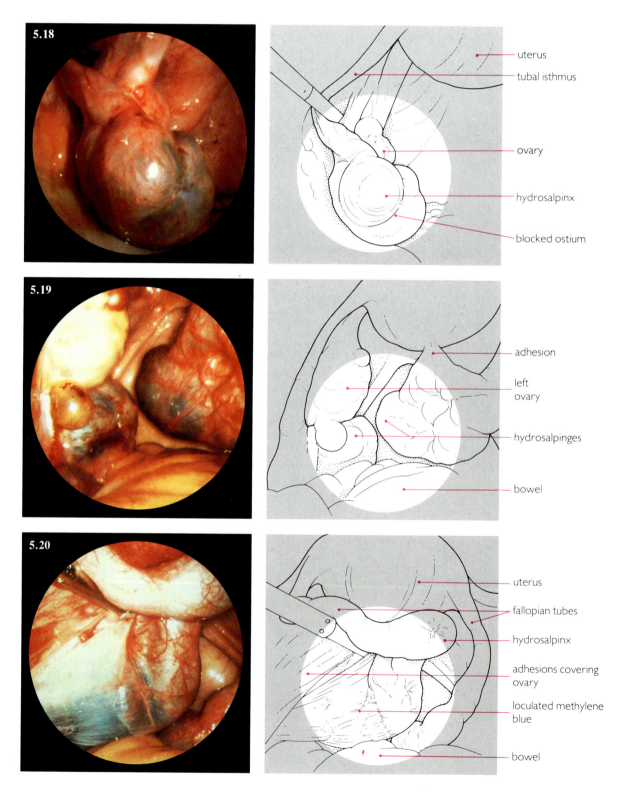

Salpingitis isthmica nodosa (Fig.5.21) is an uncommon cause of tubal blockage. There is a well defined area of thickening, about 0.5–1.0cm long at the isthmocornual junction. The tube is white and feels firm on palpation with a probe. The remainder of the tube appears normal.

Pelvic tuberculosis is rare in western Europe. It is seen as nodules studded over the surface of the tubes and uterus. The diagnosis can be confirmed by punch biopsy (Fig.5.22), but in active infection a tuboperitoneal fistula could result. As in other forms of chronic infection, adhesions form between the uterus and adjacent organs, as in Fig.5.23, where the right tube is seen to be studded with tubercles on culdoscopy.

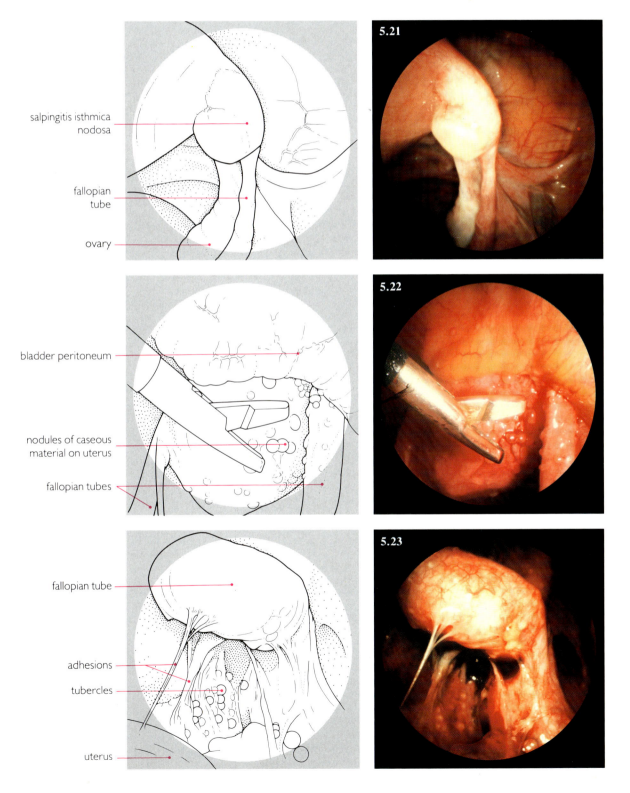

In patients with chronic pelvic inflammatory disease it is common to find lymph cysts, especially in the pouch of Douglas (Fig.5.24). These are suspended like dew-drops from the posterior surface of the uterus.

Chlamydiae are an important cause of chronic pelvic inflammatory disease, but are difficult to culture because the organisms are intracellular. The laparoscopic appearance is of chronic pelvic infection (Fig.5.25), but pus is rarely present. The coincidence of adhesions between liver and diaphragm should be remembered and the upper abdomen examined.

Equinococcal infection usually occurs in dogs, with sheep being the intermediate host. Humans occasionally contract the infection by eating contaminated food. The infection spreads from bowel to liver, resulting in formation of cysts (Fig.5.26), which may rupture and lead to intraperitoneal infection.

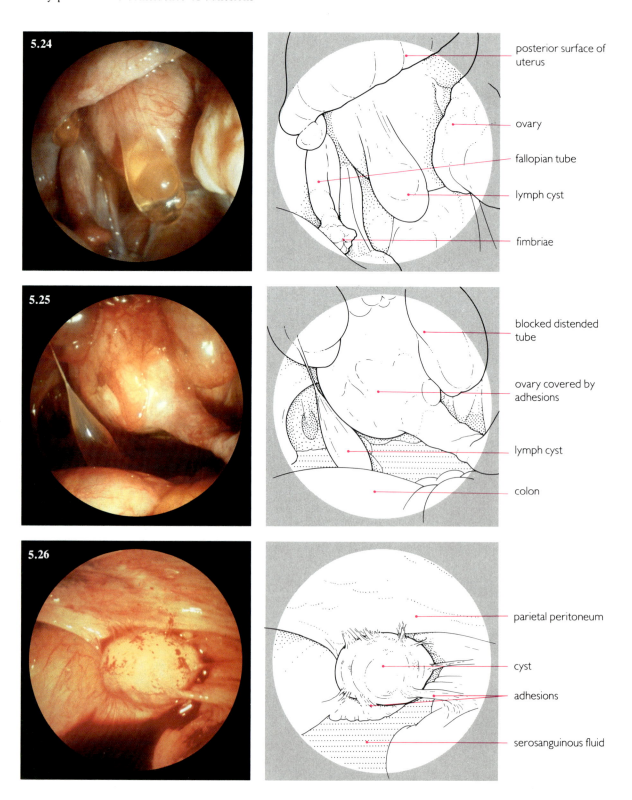

Pelvic Pain

In the patient presenting with acute pelvic pain, laparoscopy is necessary to differentiate between pelvic inflammatory disease and other causes, such as extrauterine pregnancy, appendicitis or torsion. Laparoscopy often reveals a normal pelvis but the procedure is nevertheless helpful in excluding serious intra-abdominal pathology.

Acute salpingitis (Fig.5.27) may present with clinical features similar to appendicitis (Fig.5.28) or a leaking ectopic pregnancy (Fig.5.29). Diagnostic difficulties may arise, particularly when the appendix is retrocaecal or the tubal pregnancy has not ruptured. Laparoscopy confirms the diagnosis and permits conservative medical treatment of salpingitis or a planned, cosmetic incision to remove the appendix or perform tubal surgery.

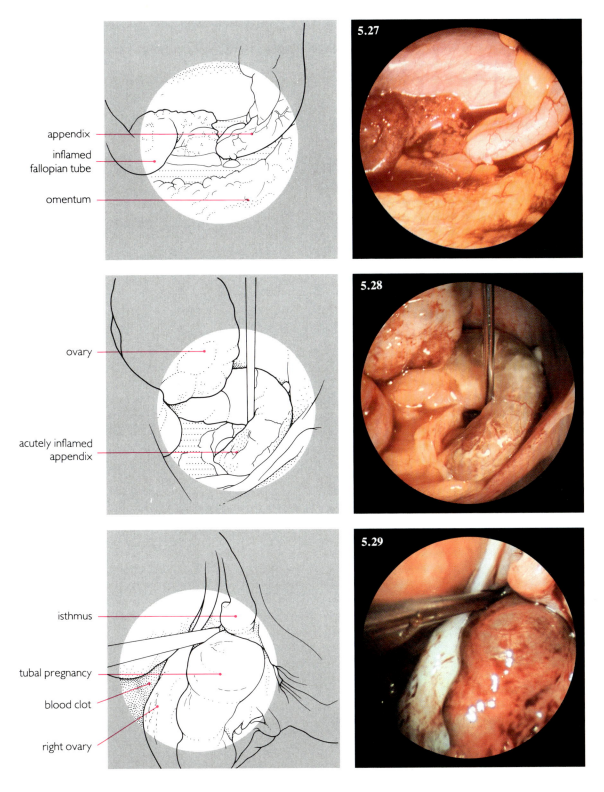

5.27

appendix
inflamed fallopian tube
omentum

5.28

ovary

acutely inflamed appendix

5.29

isthmus

tubal pregnancy

blood clot

right ovary

An endometriotic cyst causes secondary dysmenorrhoea and deep dyspareunia if it is fixed in the pouch of Douglas (Fig.5.30). If the cyst ruptures and releases altered blood into the peritoneal cavity, acute pain results, the cause of which can only be diagnosed by laparoscopy (Fig.5.31).

Endometriosis in the uterosacral ligaments may also cause deep dyspareunia. In the past, laparotomy with division of the ligaments or presacral neurectomy were performed with varying degrees of success. Endometriosis of the uterosacral ligaments can be treated by bipolar electrocoagulation (Fig.5.32), grasping the ligament and pulling it medially to avoid damaging the ureter before applying the current.

Torsion of the adnexa produces acute and severe pain. A large twisted ovarian cyst

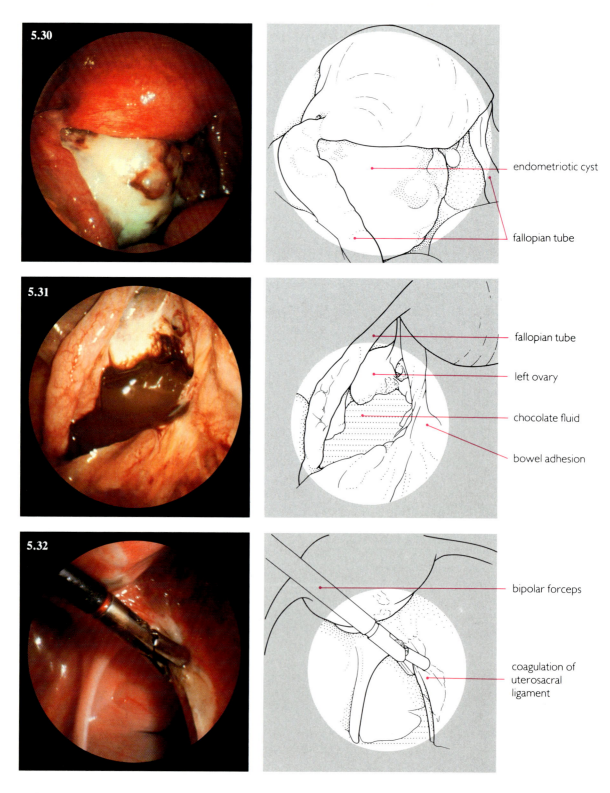

5.30 — endometriotic cyst / fallopian tube

5.31 — fallopian tube / left ovary / chocolate fluid / bowel adhesion

5.32 — bipolar forceps / coagulation of uterosacral ligament

(Fig.5.33) will often be palpable in the abdomen or in the pouch of Douglas but, even when the tumour is tender, the diagnosis may be in doubt and diverticular disease or other pelvic tumours should be excluded before proceeding to laparotomy. The blue discoloration of the ovarian cyst and the dark colour of the tube involved in the torsion are typical.

Torsion of the tube is uncommon. Even though a tube such as that in Fig.5.34 may look purple and infarcted, attempts should be made to untwist it, either laparoscopically or by laparotomy, to ascertain whether it is still viable. When a tube has undergone torsion through several revolutions (Fig.5.35), it should be removed.

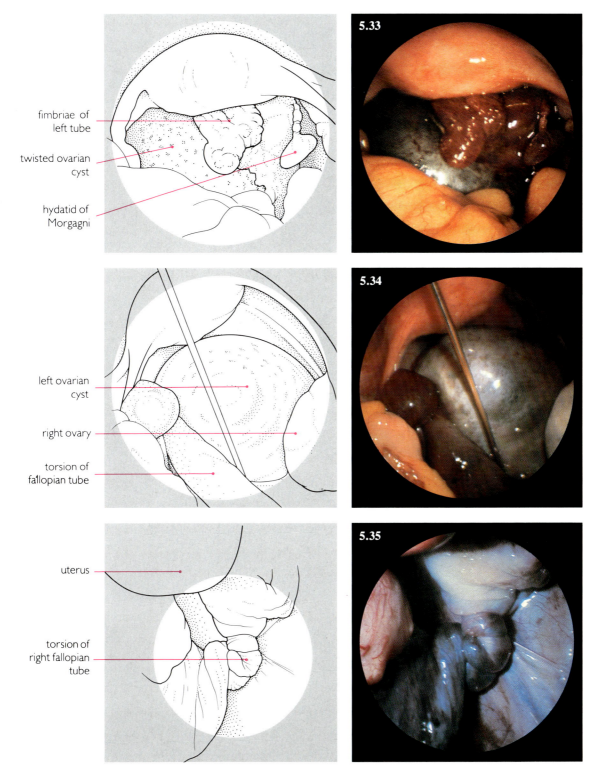

Fibroids cause pelvic pain when they undergo degeneration, torsion around a narrow pedicle or when there is bleeding from vessels on their surface. Red degeneration is common in pregnancy and should be treated conservatively. Pain from degeneration of a small subserous fibroid (Fig.5.36) rarely occurs at other times and can only be diagnosed with certainty by laparoscopy.

More dubious causes of pain are uterine retroversion and varicosities in the broad ligament or mesosalpinx (Fig.5.37). A mobile retroverted uterus (Fig.5.38) may cause deep dyspareunia, but if it is fixed in the pouch of Douglas, endometriosis or pelvic inflammatory disease should be suspected. Varicose veins are commonly seen in the broad ligament on routine examination and although it has been suggested that they can cause chronic pain, it is difficult to substantiate this claim.

Although the gynaecologist is primarily concerned with the pelvic organs, no

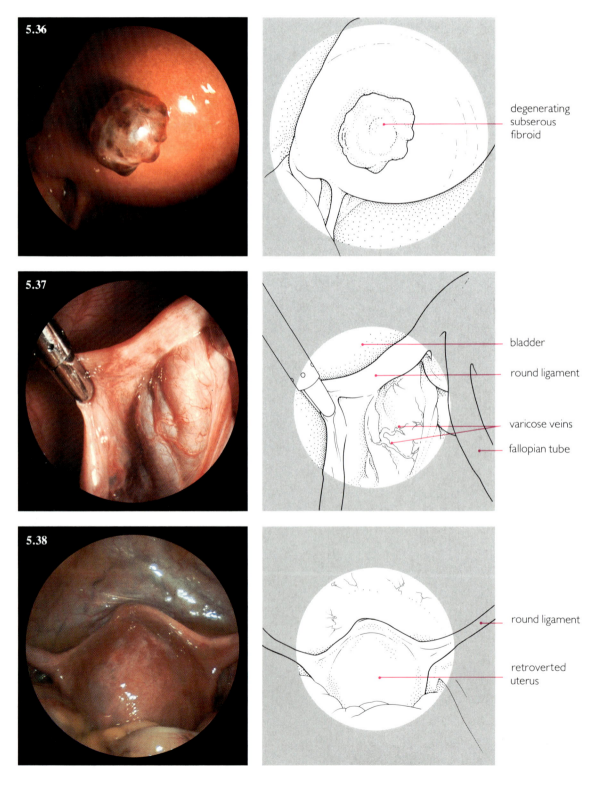

5.36 — degenerating subserous fibroid

5.37 — bladder, round ligament, varicose veins, fallopian tube

5.38 — round ligament, retroverted uterus

laparoscopy is complete without examining the remainder of the abdominal cavity. Fine adhesions (Fig.5.39) between the liver and the undersurface of the diaphragm are not significant, but more extensive adhesions (Fig.5.40), which constitute the Fitzhugh–Curtis syndrome, give rise to upper abdominal pain. These adhesions are usually avascular and can be safely divided, coagulating any that may bleed. The pain is relieved immediately. Occasionally, laparoscopy is of value in the management of acute trauma or postoperative complications by confirming the presence of a retroperitoneal haematoma (Fig.5.41). Suspected intraperitoneal bleeding or bowel damage can also be confirmed or excluded in the dangerously ill patient without resorting to laparotomy.

Reference

Sutton CJG (1986) *Lasers in Medical Science, Vol. I.* pp 25-31. London: Baillière Tindall.

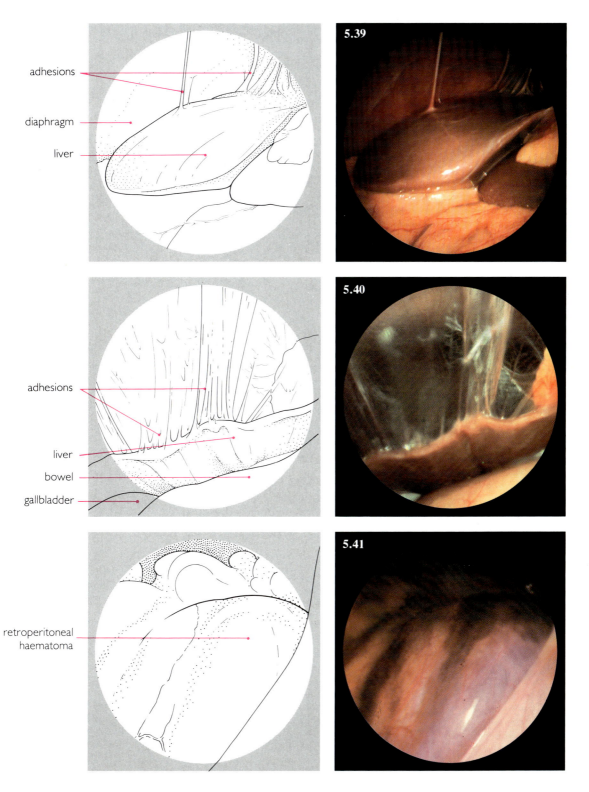

adhesions
diaphragm
liver

5.39

adhesions
liver
bowel
gallbladder

5.40

retroperitoneal haematoma

5.41

CHAPTER

6

ENDOMETRIOSIS AND PELVIC TUMOURS

Ovarian Endometriosis

The laparoscopic appearances of endometriosis show wide variation, from minimal disease with 'powder burns' to large chocolate cysts with adhesions. The clinical features may be similar to pelvic inflammatory disease, with which it can be confused. Ovarian endometriosis must also be distinguished from functional ovarian cysts and tumours, especially dermoids and pseudomucinous cysts. Small endometriotic cysts can be missed on laparoscopic examination unless a double puncture technique is used, lifting the ovary and examining both lateral and medial surfaces. A small lesion will appear well defined and black (Fig.6.1). A slightly larger endometrioma often causes puckering of the ovarian cortex (Fig.6.2). Fig.6.3 shows an endometrioma at the lower pole of the ovary with a thin-walled fimbrial cyst attached to the tube.

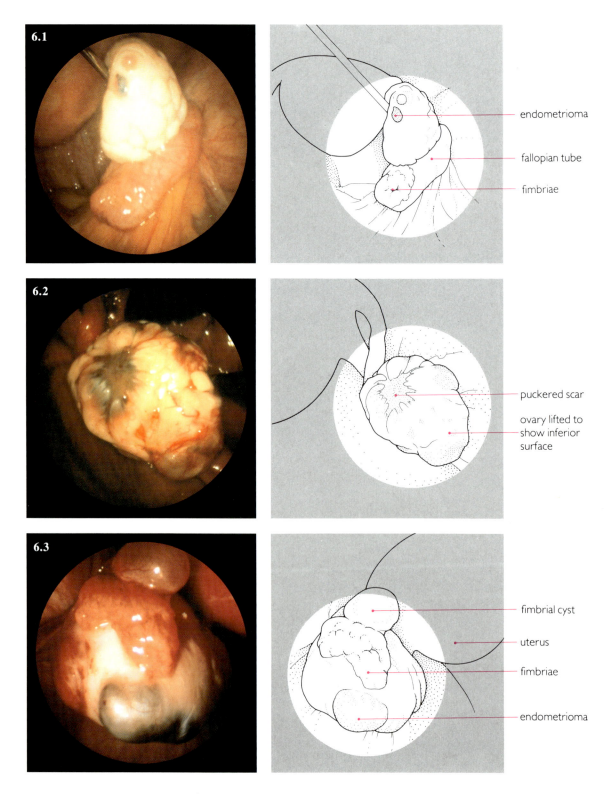

6.1
— endometrioma
— fallopian tube
— fimbriae

6.2
— puckered scar
— ovary lifted to show inferior surface

6.3
— fimbrial cyst
— uterus
— fimbriae
— endometrioma

Ovarian endometriosis is often bilateral and the ovaries may adhere in the midline, behind the body of the uterus (Fig.6.4). Even with quite extensive lesions, it is uncommon for the tubes to be blocked. As the ovaries increase in size they become less mobile and adhere to the surrounding structures such as bowel, tube, uterus and the peritoneum of the cul-de-sac. Manipulation of the ovary will often lead to rupture of the cyst with release of copious viscid, chocolate-coloured fluid into the peri-

toneal cavity (Fig.6.5). The end result of this process is gross scarring with adhesions (Fig.6.6).

Small deposits of endometriosis can be destroyed by coagulation during diagnostic laparoscopy. Larger lesions usually require laparotomy but, with experience, they can be excised endoscopically.

A large ovarian endometrioma may fill the pouch of Douglas and become densely adherent to the uterus. The tubes are stretched

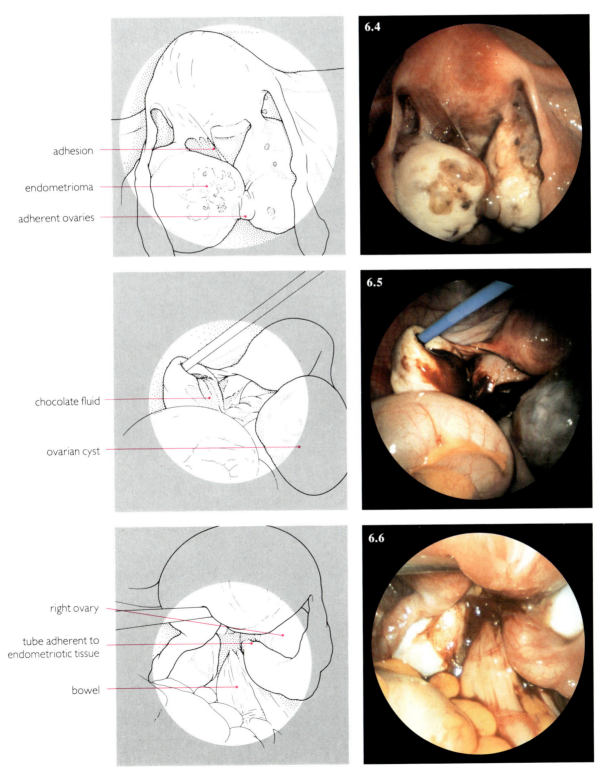

adhesion

endometrioma

adherent ovaries

chocolate fluid

ovarian cyst

right ovary

tube adherent to
endometriotic tissue

bowel

6.4

6.5

6.6

over the tumour mass. Secondary dysmenorrhoea is the main presenting symptom, but endometriomata will also cause deep dyspareunia and menorrhagia. In Fig.6.7 the condition has progressed too far for pelviscopic surgery, and such large tumours fail to resolve with suppression of menstruation by steroids or danazol therapy. Laparotomy and ovarian cystectomy are necessary, and in extensive disease, oophorectomy is the treatment of choice. Peritoneal adhesions (Fig.6.8) or fibrosis make both endoscopic surgery and laparotomy more demanding; the latter operation often requires magnification and microsurgical techniques. In Fig.6.9 a fimbrial cyst is an incidental finding in a patient with extensive endometriosis.

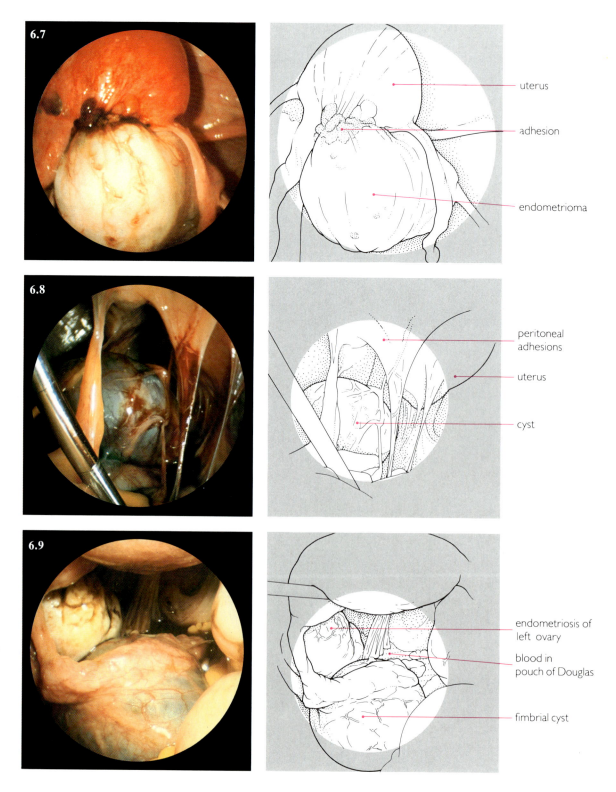

Peritoneal Endometriosis

Even small endometriotic deposits can cause severe symptoms, while large lesions may not cause pain. Apart from the ovary, the most common site for small deposits is the peritoneum of the pouch of Douglas and the uterosacral ligaments (Fig.6.10). Small lesions can easily be missed. The telescope should be advanced into the pelvis until the lens almost touches the endometrioma; fine details can then be examined. The characteristic black appearance is easily distinguished from the surrounding blood vessels and petechial haemorrhages in the peritoneum (Fig.6.11). These lesions can be treated by laser, which vaporizes the tissue, leaving no residue and little scarring (Fig.6.12). Alternatively, treatment with danazol or progestogens will prevent further bleeding into the deposits and aid healing.

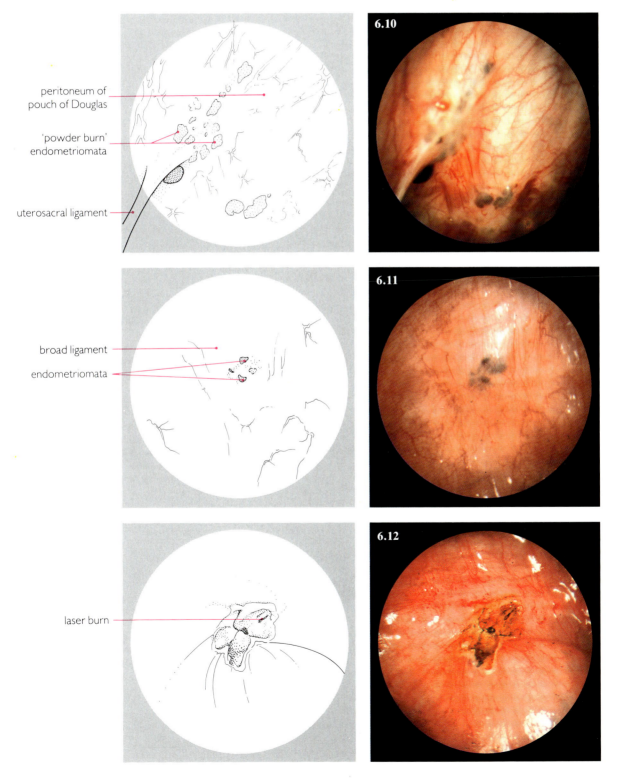

Endometriosis often develops on the uterosacral ligament, and occasionally it may be superficial to major structures such as the external iliac vessel or the ureter.

Endometriotic spots can also be destroyed by application of heat using a low-voltage current from the Endocoagulator (Figs.6.13 & 6.14) or by bipolar diathermy (Fig.6.15). The foot pedal should be depressed only when the point is in contact with the deposit. As the current is applied, the lesion first bubbles and then turns white in colour. Scar tissue soon forms and the patient's symptoms are relieved. Unipolar electrocoagulation should not be used because of the danger of burning surrounding tissues. Suppression of menstruation by danazol or progestogens can be used as an alternative or adjunct to thermal coagulation.

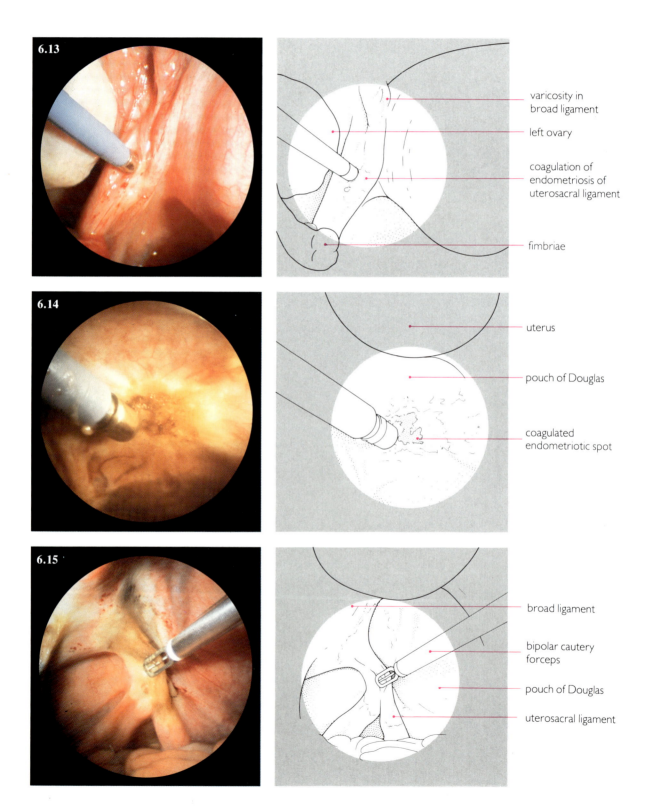

6.13
- varicosity in broad ligament
- left ovary
- coagulation of endometriosis of uterosacral ligament
- fimbriae

6.14
- uterus
- pouch of Douglas
- coagulated endometriotic spot

6.15
- broad ligament
- bipolar cautery forceps
- pouch of Douglas
- uterosacral ligament

Another common site of pelvic endo-metriosis is the uterovesical fold of peritoneum (Fig.6.16). This can cause severe urinary symptoms including cyclical dysuria and pelvic pain and, less frequently, cyclical haematuria. Treatment by surgical excision and hormones is preferable to high-voltage diathermy because of the danger of damage to the bladder. An endometrioma of the uterine fundus (Fig.6.17) is very obvious. Adeno-myosis deep in the myometrium cannot be seen with the laparoscope.

Endometriosis of the Fallopian Tube
It is rare to find endometriosis in the fallopian tube. In Fig.6.18 a small endometrioma on the antemesenteric border is causing distortion.

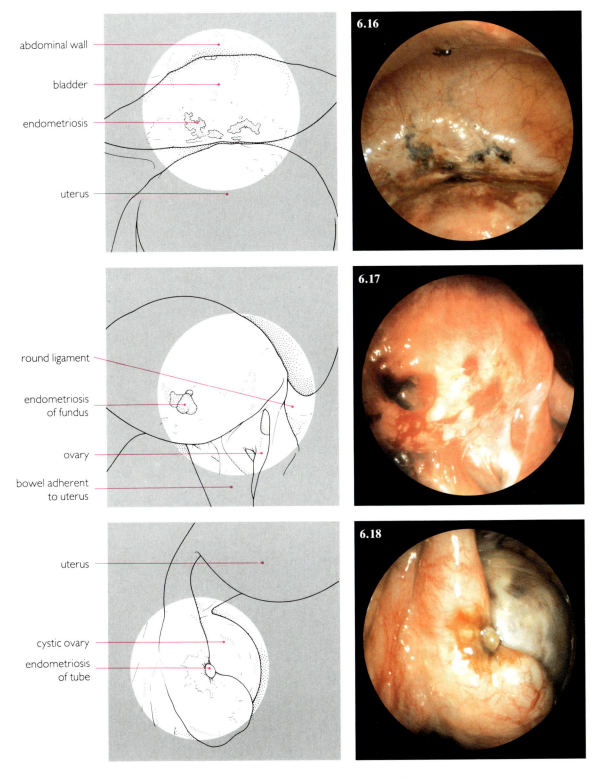

6.7

In Fig.6.19 a larger endometrioma is present on the ampulla of the tube causing a lesser degree of distortion. This could be treated by microsurgical excision or danazol. Rarely, the appendix may become adherent to an endometriotic nodule on the tube (Fig.6.20). Appendectomy with excision of the area of endometriosis should be performed.

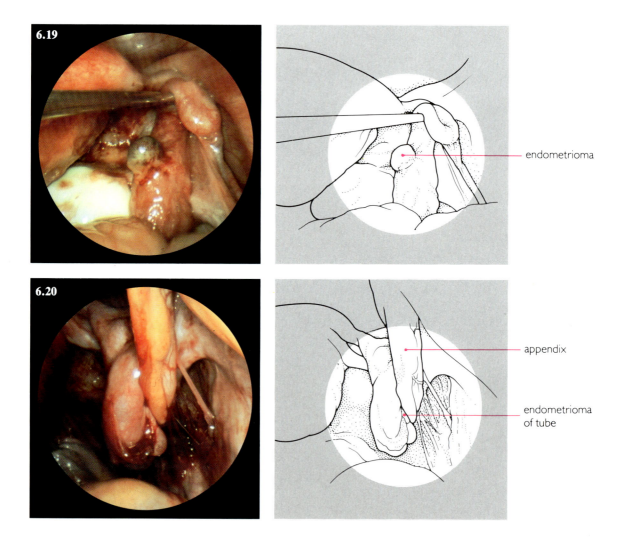

endometrioma

appendix

endometrioma
of tube

Fibroids

Fibroids and endometriosis commonly occur together and may be encountered as an incidental finding at laparoscopy. Large fibroids are usually obvious on clinical examination, but small ones are often unsuspected. A small subserous fibroid is usually insignificant when in the fundus (Fig.6.21), but if close to the intramural portion of the tube it can be a cause of tubal infertility.

Differentiation from an ovarian tumour, either clinically or by ultrasound, may be difficult. Pelvic examination will detect either a large pedunculated fundal fibroid (Fig.6.22) or one occupying the pouch of Douglas (Fig.6.23), but laparoscopy is required to determine the exact pathology.

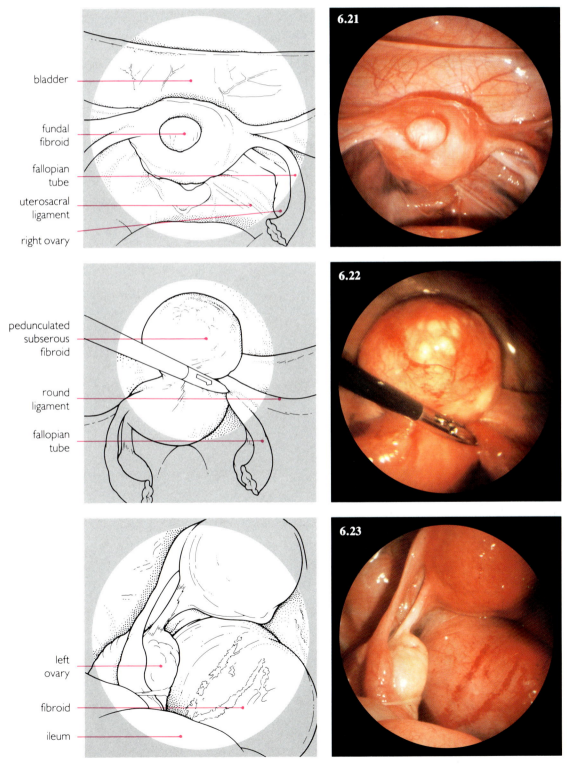

6.21

bladder

fundal fibroid

fallopian tube

uterosacral ligament

right ovary

pedunculated subserous fibroid

round ligament

fallopian tube

6.22

left ovary

fibroid

ileum

6.23

A cornual fibroid may be mistaken for a bicornuate uterus, even at laparoscopy. In Fig.6.24 there is one anterior wall fibroid with a second one distorting the intramural portion of the tube. Methylene blue injected through the cervix has been intravasated because the tube is blocked by external pressure. Surgery to remove this fibroid must avoid the lumen of the tube.

Multiple intramural fibroids (Fig.6.25) grossly distort the uterus, but even large tumours are compatible with pregnancy unless the tube is distorted or blocked.

Microfibromata on the ovary (Fig.6.26) are usually of little importance; rarely, they may slowly enlarge and eventually cause Meigs' syndrome with ascites and a pleural effusion.

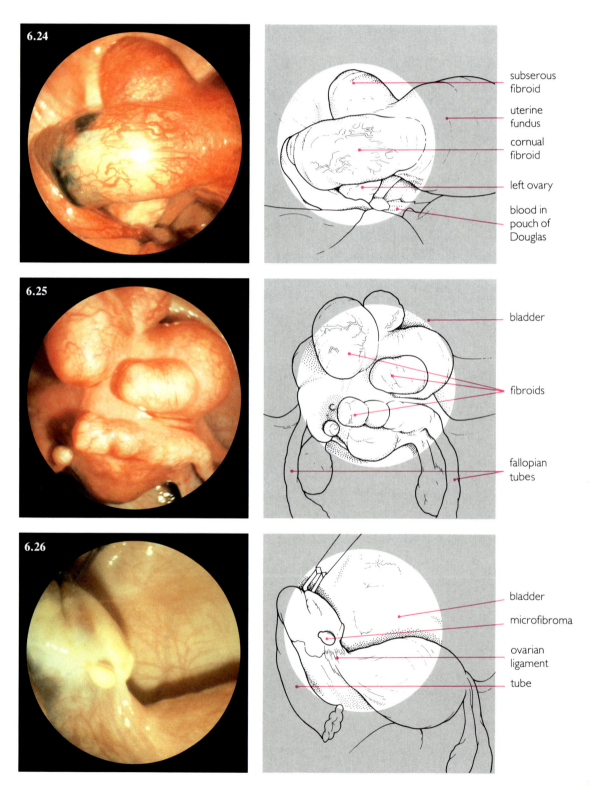

Myomectomy

Generally, myomectomy requires laparotomy and enucleation of the fibroids. This is necessary if the fibroid is intramural, but if it is subserous and pedunculated (Fig.6.27), it is possible to remove it laparoscopically. The pedicle is first coagulated with crocodile forceps (Fig.6.28) and then divided with large scissors; any bleeding vessels are treated with a point coagulator. Finally, the fibroid is removed by morcellement and peritoneal lavage is perfomed (Fig.6.29).

Polypoid submucous fibroids can be removed by blind curettage or, more precisely, with hysteroscopically directed forceps.

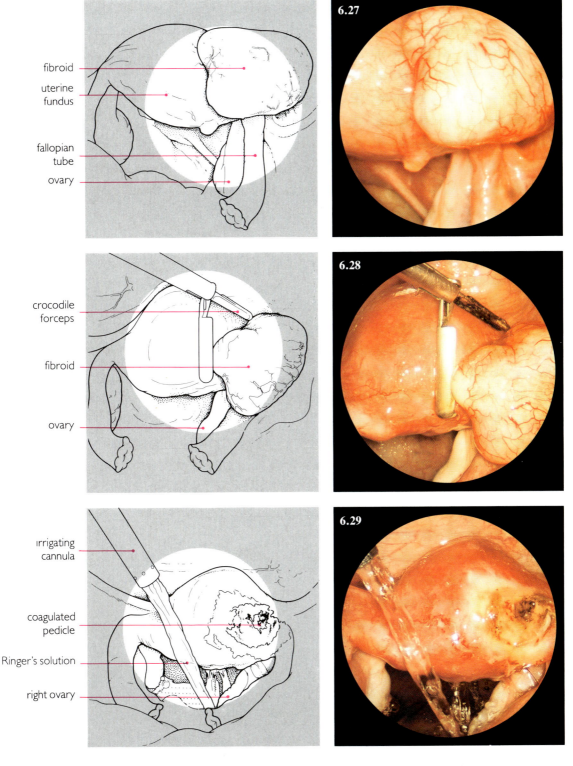

6.27

fibroid
uterine fundus
fallopian tube
ovary

6.28

crocodile forceps
fibroid
ovary

6.29

irrigating cannula
coagulated pedicle
Ringer's solution
right ovary

Physiological Ovarian Cysts

It may be difficult to differentiate between endometriosis, fibroids and ovarian cysts without the use of laparoscopy. Physiological cysts in the ovary vary in size at different phases in the menstrual cycle. The dominant Graafian follicle enlarges in the pre-ovulatory phase to reach a diameter of 20–25mm (Fig.6.30). After ovulation, the corpus luteum may achieve a similar size (Fig.6.31). Laparoscopy or ultrasound will reveal these cysts, but they are usually undetectable on pelvic examination. There can be intraperitoneal bleeding at ovulation, or the follicle may rupture, both of which cause pain and require laparoscopy to distinguish them from ectopic pregnancy. Occasionally, especially with the use of drugs to induce ovulation, the cysts may enlarge even more and must then be differentiated from other pelvic tumours.

Small fimbrial cysts are common and normal

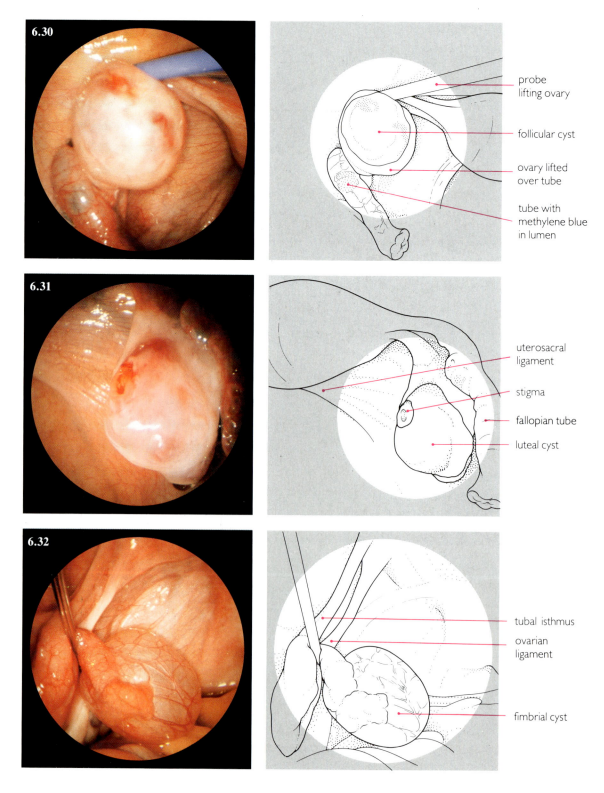

6.30
probe lifting ovary
follicular cyst
ovary lifted over tube
tube with methylene blue in lumen

6.31
uterosacral ligament
stigma
fallopian tube
luteal cyst

6.32
tubal isthmus
ovarian ligament
fimbrial cyst

(Fig.6.32); they are never clinically relevant unless they undergo torsion.

Benign cystic tumours are common after puberty. They are usually found in the pouch of Douglas, displacing the uterus forwards and upwards (Fig.6.33). However, dermoid cysts often lie anterior to the uterus.

Complications of Ovarian Cysts
The fallopian tube becomes stretched over the surface of the cyst as it increases in size or, occasionally, the cyst may grow into the broad ligament, Benign cysts are usually freely mobile with no adhesions, but if there is leakage of irritant fluid contents or infection, adhesions may form (Fig.6.34). The cyst wall becomes densely adherent to the tube and the posterior surface of the uterus or, rarely, the appendix may become adherent to a spot of endometriosis on the ovary or tube (Fig.6.35).

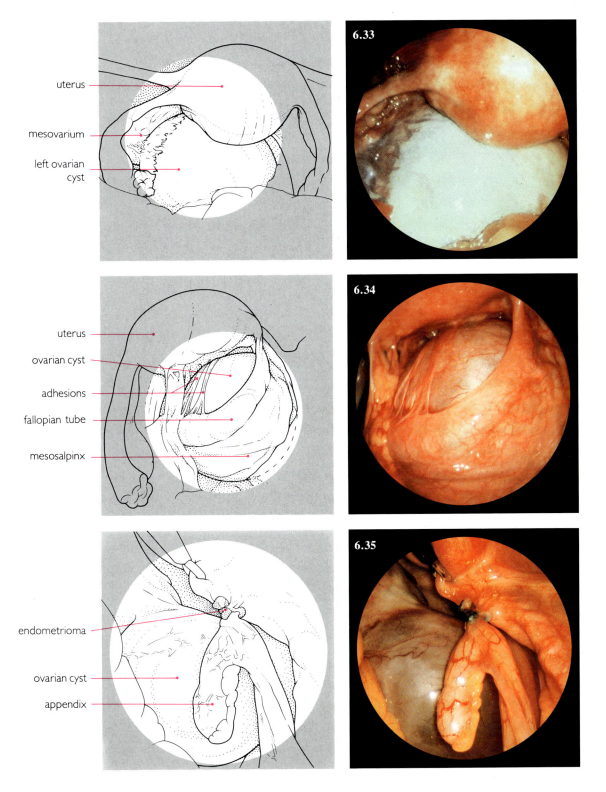

Larger cysts frequently expand into the abdomen, where they become palpable. Laparoscopy (Fig.6.36) is helpful in assessing the nature of the cyst and its relationship to surrounding structures. Treatment by laparotomy or operative laparoscopy can then be planned.

Even at laparoscopy it may be difficult to be certain of the nature of an ovarian cyst (Fig.6.37), but manipulation with a probe

leading to spillage of chocolate fluid (Fig.6.38) into the peritoneum confirms the diagnosis of endometriosis. There may be other endometriotic lesions in the contralateral ovary, uterosacral ligaments or pouch of Douglas.

Some serous cystadenomata may grow to a considerable size without causing symptoms and are only found on routine examination.

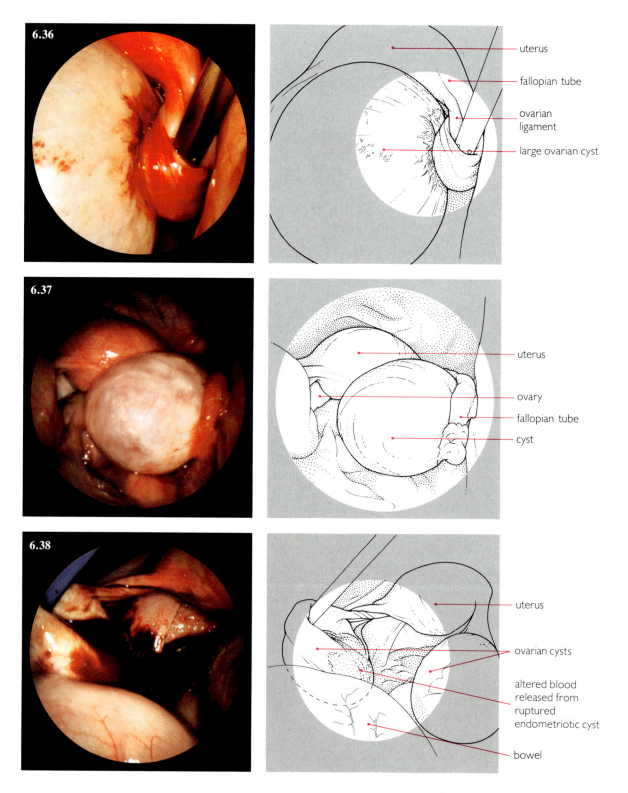

Others present with acute pain, which may be caused by torsion or sudden haemorrhage into the cyst. If this occurs, the patient will also have a palpable tender swelling in the pelvis or abdomen and there may be guarding and rigidity. Laparoscopy prior to laparotomy confirms the diagnosis and distinguishes torsion from tubal pregnancy or acute infection. There is characteristic blue discoloration of the cyst caused by haemorrhage when the venous return is obstructed (Fig.6.39). Sometimes the tube and ovary are both involved in the torsion (Fig.6.40). Cysts in the mesosalpinx (Fig.6.41) are usually small, but occasionally enlarge and become liable to torsion.

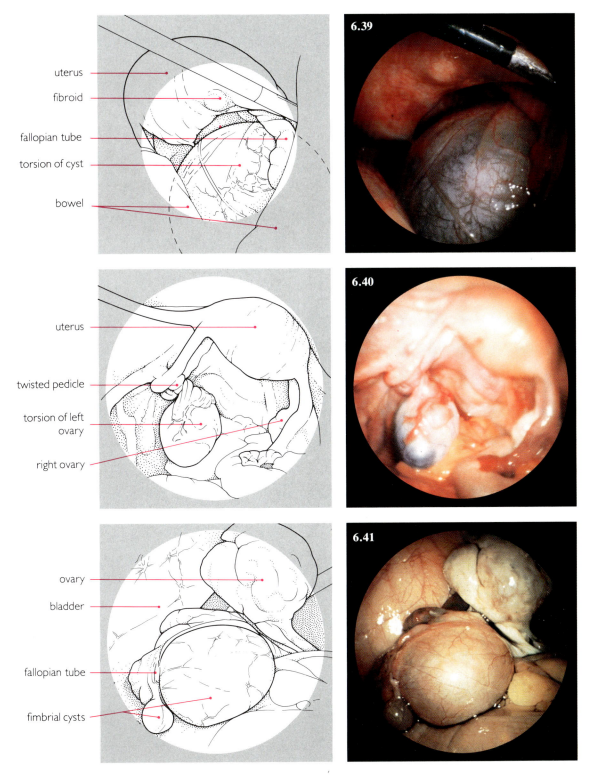

Treatment of Ovarian Cysts

Most gynaecologists will perform laparotomy to remove ovarian cysts; this must be done when there is a suspicion of malignancy. However, laparoscopic surgery can be used to aspirate and remove simple cysts.

Simple follicular cysts can be aspirated (Fig.6.42), the cyst cavity opened (Fig.6.43) and any small bleeding points in the cyst wall treated with bipolar electrocoagulation (Fig.6.44). This gives good results in simple cysts, but if the tumour is a serous or pseudo-mucinous cystadenoma and the lining is not completely removed, the opening in the capsule will close and the cyst will recur.

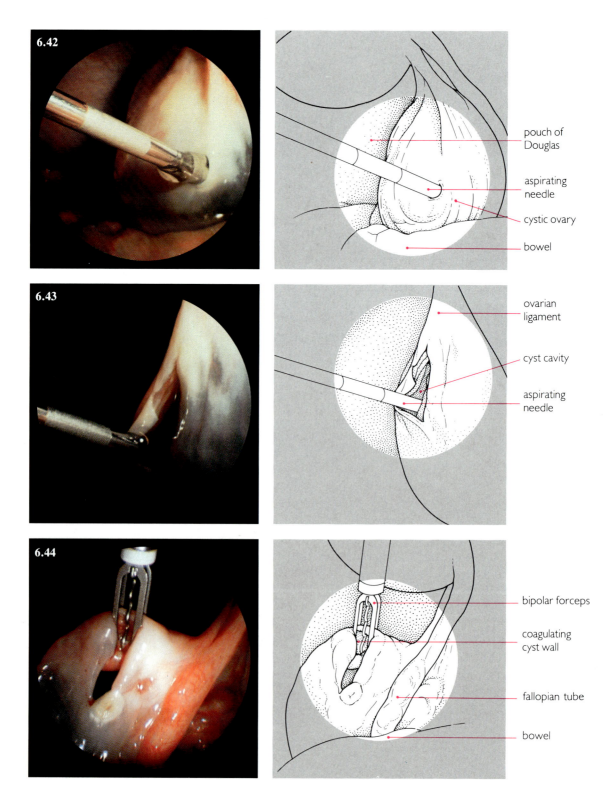

It is preferable to remove the cyst completely. First, its contents are aspirated (Fig.6.45) and the fluid is saved for cytological examination. The empty capsule is elevated (Fig.6.46) and the wall of the cyst is dissected from the ovary using forceps and scissors (Fig.6.47). The tumour is removed from the pelvis with grasping forceps through a 10mm cannula.

The surgeon has a choice of methods for treating the raw area of the ovary. It can be coagulated with bipolar diathermy or endo-coagulation. This ensures haemostasis but leaves an area of ovary to which bowel could become adherent. The risk of this can be reduced by instilling a solution of 0.5% hydro-cortisone in normal saline.

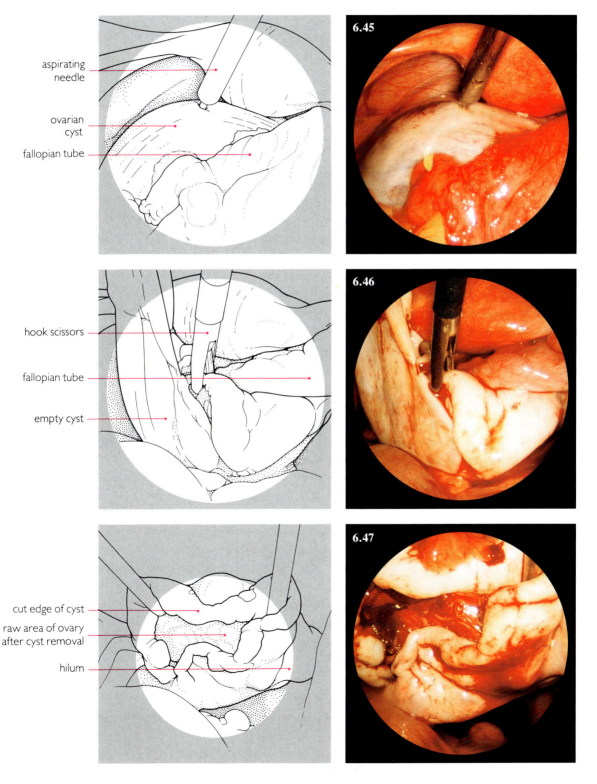

aspirating needle

ovarian cyst

fallopian tube

6.45

hook scissors

fallopian tube

empty cyst

6.46

cut edge of cyst

raw area of ovary after cyst removal

hilum

6.47

Alternatively, the ovary can be sutured, either using a needle and catgut, or by ligating the ovarian capsule with a Roeder loop (Fig.6.48).

There is always some blood in the pelvis at completion of the operation. This is washed out with Ringer's solution (Fig.6.49), using up to 3–4 litres if necessary. After multiple washes the pelvis is free of blood and a solution of hydrocortisone is instilled. Adhesions are less common after laparoscopic surgery because intestinal stasis, which is implicated in adhesion formation, does not occur, as the patient is able to eat on the evening of the operation.

A simple dermoid cyst (Fig.6.50) is removed in the same way. The liquid fatty material is aspirated. Hair and other solid tissue is removed with forceps and suction. Lavage is repeated until the pelvis is clean.

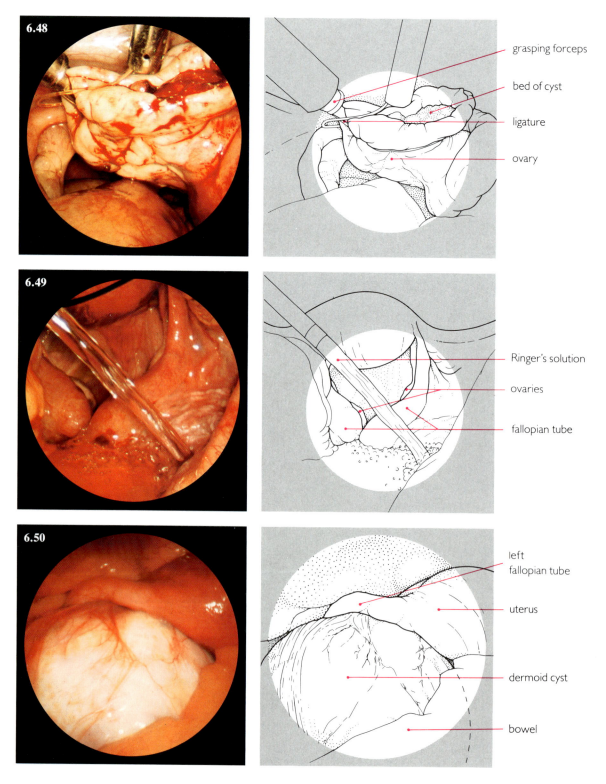

Malignant Disease

Laparoscopy or laparotomy may be the only ways to distinguish ovarian cancer from other pelvic tumours. Ultrasound can differentiate between solid and cystic masses, but laparoscopy allows precise assessment of the growth, permits tissue biopsy and enables secondary deposits in the bowel and liver to be seen, and fluid to be aspirated for cytology if ascites is present.

In the presence of extensive disease, laparoscopy must be performed with care because of the risk of bowel damage, but the procedure is valuable when the tumour is confined to the pelvis. Malignant growths are usually solid, bilateral, fixed and lobulated in appearance (Fig.6.51). Figs.6.52 and 6.53 illustrate the similarity in appearance between a hyperstimulated ovary and an ovary with carcinoma.

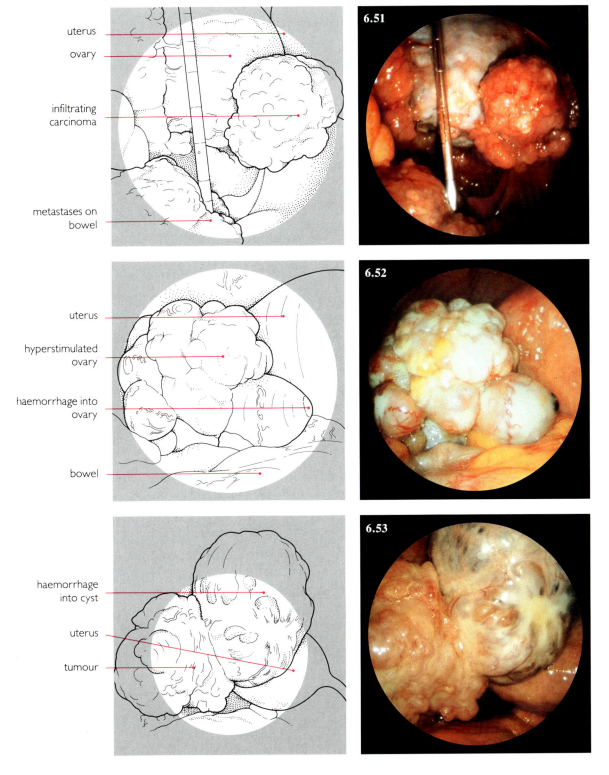

uterus

ovary

infiltrating carcinoma

metastases on bowel

6.51

uterus

hyperstimulated ovary

haemorrhage into ovary

bowel

6.52

haemorrhage into cyst

uterus

tumour

6.53

When carcinoma of the ovary is confirmed at laparoscopy, the abdominal cavity should be systematically examined for secondary deposits. The pelvis is inspected first, followed by the upper abdomen, the upper surface of the liver, the anterior surface of the gallbladder and the inferior surface of the diaphragm and the lower ribs. The secondary deposits may be single (Fig.6.54) or multiple (Fig.6.55) and are often small and discrete, but unfortunately it is a frequent finding that the liver and diaphragm are already the sites of massive deposits (Fig.6.56).

Laparoscopy is of value in determining the response to chemotherapy using a second-look procedure, but open laparotomy allows a more

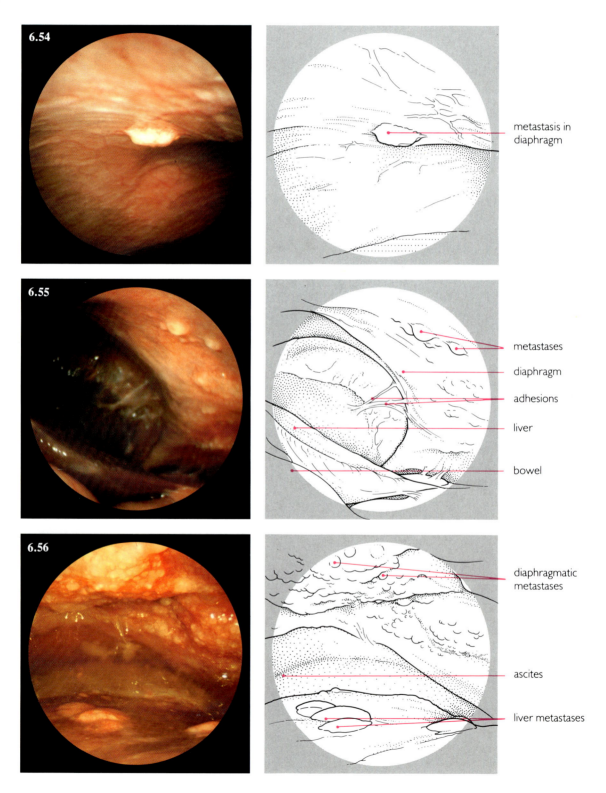

detailed examination of the abdomen and retroperitoneal nodes. Figs.6.57 and 6.58 show a subdiaphragmatic secondary which was biopsied prior to treatment with cis-platinum. Following this, a second laparoscopy was performed; the tumour deposit was smaller (Fig.6.59) and histology showed no active cancer cells but merely fibroblasts and muscle (Fig.6.60).

The value of the second-look procedure is that chemotherapy can be given in a more controlled manner; the treatment can be recommenced if there is any evidence of activity in the tumour.

Secondary deposits are seen not only in the liver and inferior surface of the diaphragm but also on the parietal peritoneum, omentum and

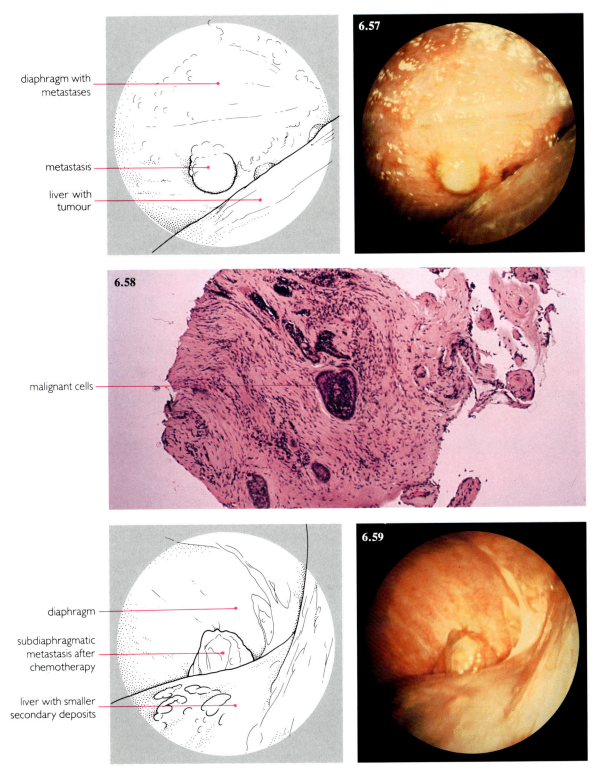

diaphragm with metastases

metastasis

liver with tumour

6.57

6.58

malignant cells

diaphragm

subdiaphragmatic metastasis after chemotherapy

liver with smaller secondary deposits

6.59

bowel. Peritoneal deposits can be biopsied (Fig.6.61), but there is a risk that a skin or subcutaneous deposit may develop if the biopsy forceps pass through a parietal metastasis.

Care must be taken when the secondary is close to bowel (Fig.6.62) as the latter could be damaged by biopsy. There should be no difficulty in distinguishing a tumour deposit from an appendix epiploica, but problems in

taking a biopsy may occur when the metastasis invades the bowel wall. Bleeding from the biopsy site cannot be easily controlled by diathermy, and injury to the mucosa requires laparotomy and primary suture. Direct bowel injury by the trocar is possible at second-look laparoscopy if the gut is adherent to the abdominal wall.

It may sometimes be difficult to differentiate primary bowel tumours from secondary de-

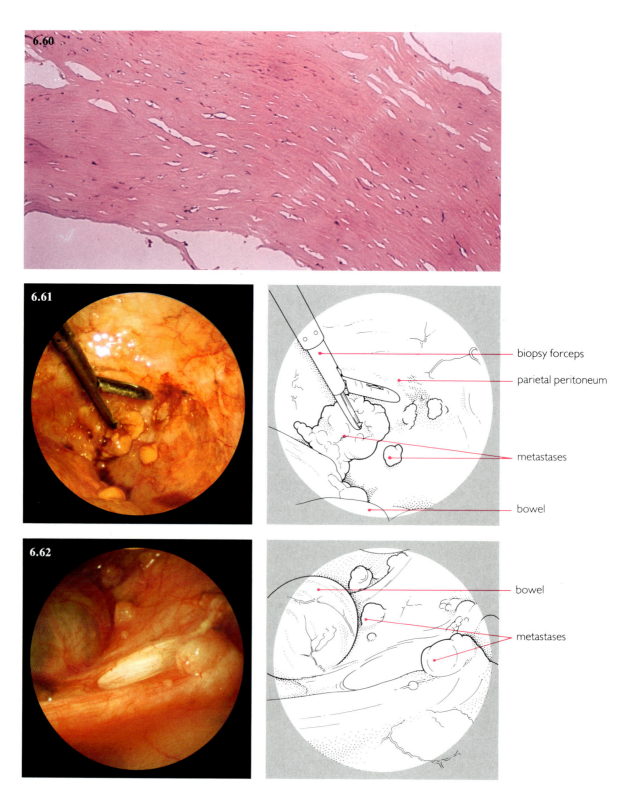

posits because the surface of the large bowel is frequently studded with metastases from ovarian carcinoma (Fig.6.63). A primary tumour of descending or sigmoid colon (Figs.6.64 & 6.65) may be mistaken for carcinoma of the left ovary on palpation. Barium studies, sigmoidoscopy or colonoscopy with biopsy should confirm the diagnosis and the extent of the disease. If ovarian carcinoma is suspected, ultrasound and laparoscopy should be performed. If a growth is found in the bowel at diagnostic laparoscopy, both ovaries should be inspected to exclude primary carcinoma or a Kruckenberg tumour.

Primary carcinoma of the tube (Fig.6.66) is rare and can only be diagnosed by endoscopic examination and biopsy or by laparotomy. It should not be confused with metastatic spread from carcinoma of the ovary.

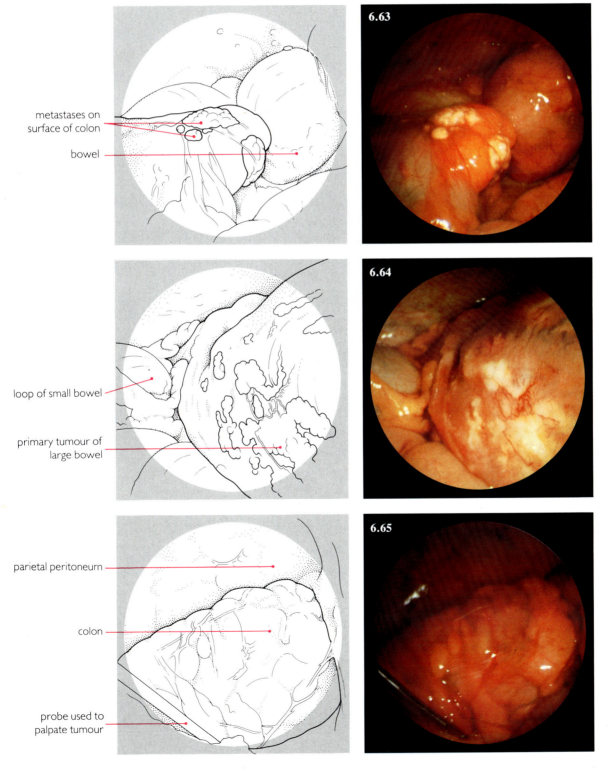

Metastatic cancer in the omentum can produce a solitary tumour or a thickened, nodular mass (Fig.6.67). Biopsy is usually easy but may be accompanied by brisk bleeding, which must be controlled by coagulation or endoligature. This is difficult if the deposits are large or close to the abdominal wall.

Ovarian carcinoma rarely infiltrates bone, even in the terminal stages of the disease, but this complication may be suspected if pain is the dominant symptom. Radiographs or bone scans will usually demonstrate the deposits, and endoscopy has little place in these circumstances. However, a superficial bony deposit in the pelvis or sacrum can sometimes be seen in a thin patient. A secondary deposit in the lower rib cage (Fig.6.68) is more obvious.

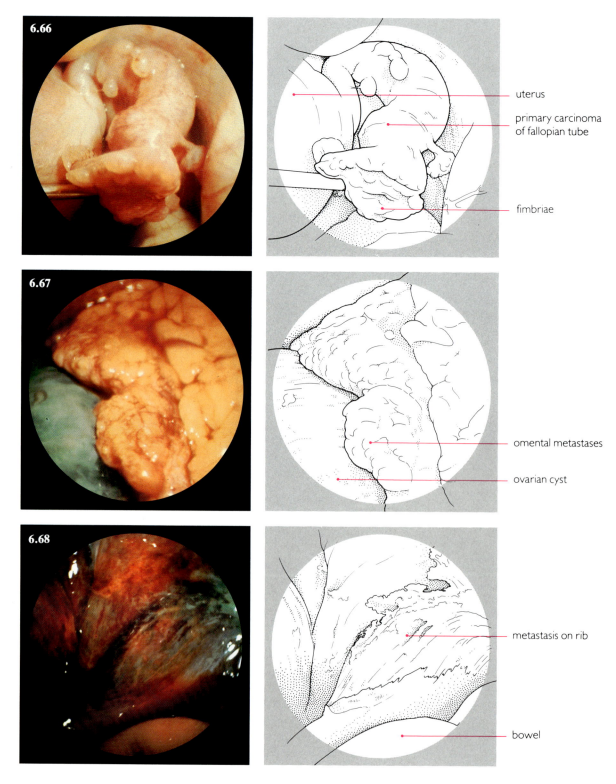

6.66

uterus

primary carcinoma of fallopian tube

fimbriae

6.67

omental metastases

ovarian cyst

6.68

metastasis on rib

bowel

It must always be remembered that laparoscopy is an invasive technique which disturbs tissue planes and can lead to direct spread of tumour cells. It is possible for a patient to develop metastases in the umbilicus (Fig.6.69) at the site of insertion of the trocar.

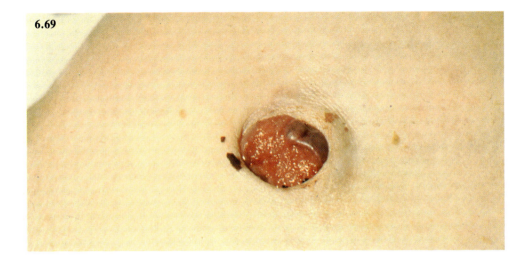

6.69

CHAPTER

7

STERILIZATION

Laparoscopic sterilization is the most frequently performed endoscopic operation. The advantages over other procedures are that the incisions are small, the duration of stay is hospital is short, and postoperative recovery is rapid.

Coagulation

In the classical method of unipolar electro-coagulation, laparoscopy is performed through a standard umbilical incision. A trocar is inserted through a second suprapubic or iliac fossa incision and Palmer biopsy forceps are introduced into the abdomen. As in all sterilization operations, the tube must be positively identified by seeing its full length, including the fimbriae. The isthmus is grasped and an electric current is passed through the tube until it bubbles and collapses. It can then be divided by advancing the sheath of the forceps so that the cutting edge transects the tube (Fig.7.1). Alternatively, it can be cut with hook scissors.

The disadvantages of this operation are the excessive heat production and the amount of local tissue destruction, which makes reconstructive surgery more difficult. Further heat may be transmitted directly along tissue planes and cause burns a short distance from the operation site. Even more serious complications may occur as the current returns through the body to the diathermy plate and thence to the generator. Electric burns can be produced outside the visual field of the surgeon, and cause damage to the bowel and other structures (Fig.7.2). Moreover, if the laparoscope sheath comes into contact with the electric forceps, the patient's skin and the operator may be burnt.

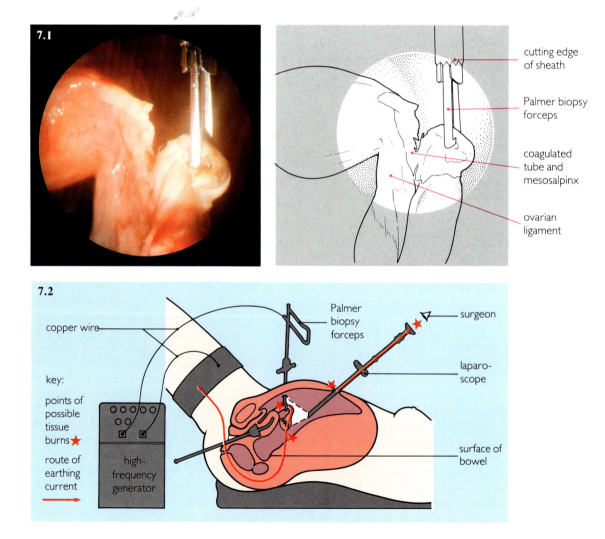

7.1

cutting edge of sheath

Palmer biopsy forceps

coagulated tube and mesosalpinx

ovarian ligament

7.2

copper wire

Palmer biopsy forceps

surgeon

laparo-scope

key:

points of possible tissue burns ★

route of earthing current →

high-frequency generator

surface of bowel

As these complications can lead to serious injury or death, other safer procedures have been developed. In bipolar electrocoagulation the tube is grasped with forceps as before (Fig.7.3), but the electric current passes from one blade of the forceps to the other (Fig.7.4). There is no significant spread of heat from the operation site and no risk of electric burns outside the operation field, although the forceps must still not be allowed to touch the bowel and a gas which does not support combustion must be used.

The tube can be divided with scissors (Fig.7.5), or a segment of tube between the coagulated sites can be removed with biopsy forceps for histological confirmation. This may increase the possibility of fistula formation and of pregnancy, but it provides medicolegal proof that the operation has been performed correctly.

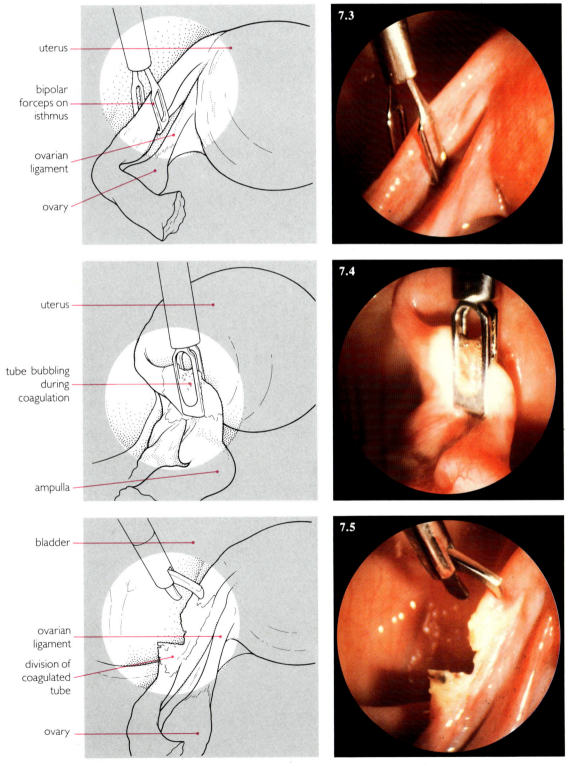

7.3

7.4

7.5

uterus
bipolar forceps on isthmus
ovarian ligament
ovary

uterus
tube bubbling during coagulation
ampulla

bladder
ovarian ligament
division of coagulated tube
ovary

Endocoagulation uses a low-voltage current to apply heat at 100°C to the tube between the blades of crocodile forceps (Fig 7.6). This is not only safer than other electrical methods, but also, if local anaesthetic is used, is less painful.

The tubal isthmus is grasped with the forceps (Fig.7.7) and controlled heat applied for 30 seconds. The process is repeated until approximately 2cm of tube has been coagulated. This segment is divided with hook scissors (Fig.7.8) and the cut end coagulated again with forceps or a point coagulator. Timing is confirmed by an audible signal from the generator, so that the surgeon is able to watch the tube being coagulated without lifting his eye from the laparoscope.

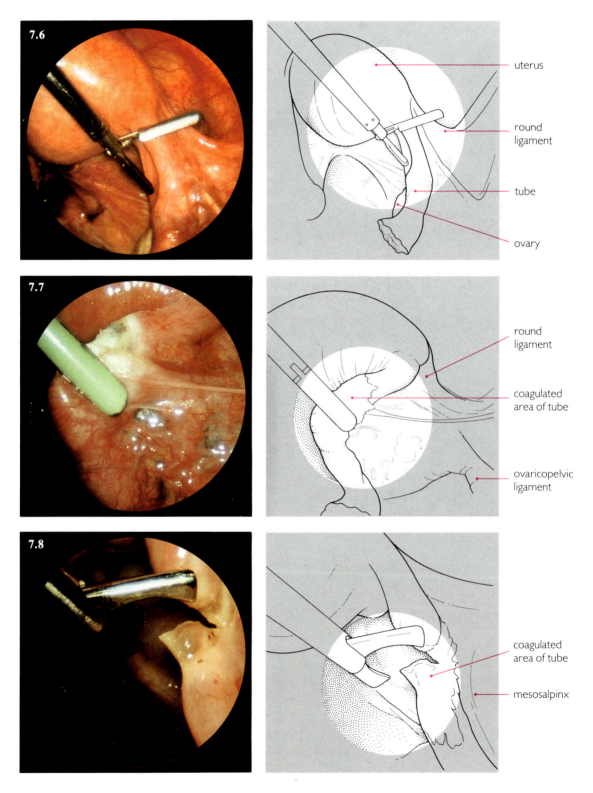

7.6

uterus
round ligament
tube
ovary

7.7

round ligament
coagulated area of tube
ovaricopelvic ligament

7.8

coagulated area of tube
mesosalpinx

Operations using electrocoagulation are potentially dangerous. There have been many serious complications caused by burns to bowel and other organs and mishaps of this type have, in certain cases, led to subsequent legal action against the surgeon involved.

Mechanical Blockage

When the dangers of electrocoagulation began to be appreciated in the early 1970s, a number of mechanical methods of tubal obstruction were developed. Some of these were initially designed for minilaparotomy and later modified for laparoscopy.

The main advantage of mechanical obstruction of the tube is that there is no risk of burns, since no heat is being used. There is also less tissue destruction because the clip occludes only a small segment of tube, making reversal of sterilization easier and more likely to be successful.

The first clips to be used were simple haemostats, which proved to be too weak and tended to fracture at the hinge. Four types of clips are currently available (Fig.7.9); these are usually applied through a second incision, either suprapubically or lateral to the umbilicus. In the latter case, the incision must avoid the inferior epigastric artery, which can be seen by transilluminating the abdominal wall.

The Hulka clip, the most commonly used type, is made of plastic with a gold-plated steel spring. The clip applicator (Fig.7.10) is

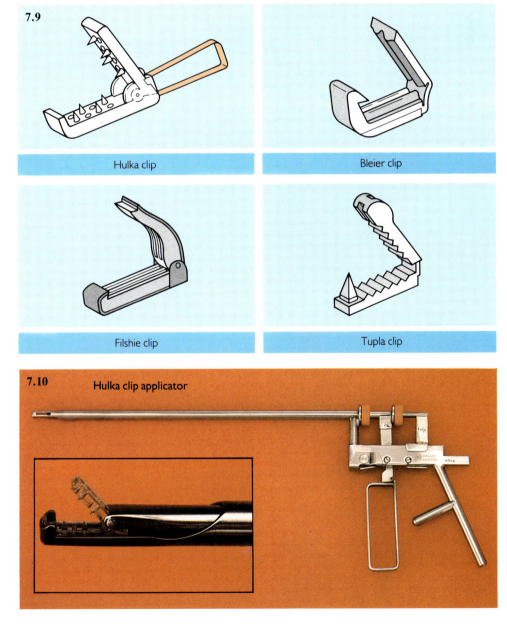

7.9

Hulka clip

Bleier clip

Filshie clip

Tupla clip

7.10 Hulka clip applicator

inserted through a second incision. The full diameter of the tube is grasped at the isthmus (Fig.7.11) and the jaws of the clip closed (Fig.7.12). The spring is pushed fowards until it locks and the clip is then released from the applicator (Fig.7.13).

Postoperatively, the patient may complain of colicky lower abdominal pain, which may last for up to three days as the clip crushes the tube.

In our experience of 3000 Hulka clip sterilizations, 15 intrauterine and one ectopic pregnancy occurred. This failure rate can be further reduced by applying two clips close together on each tube. We have not had a single case of pregnancy following interval sterilization since the technique was altered in 1981. However, clip sterilization carried out simultaneously with termination of pregnancy does carry a greater risk of failure because the tubes are thicker.

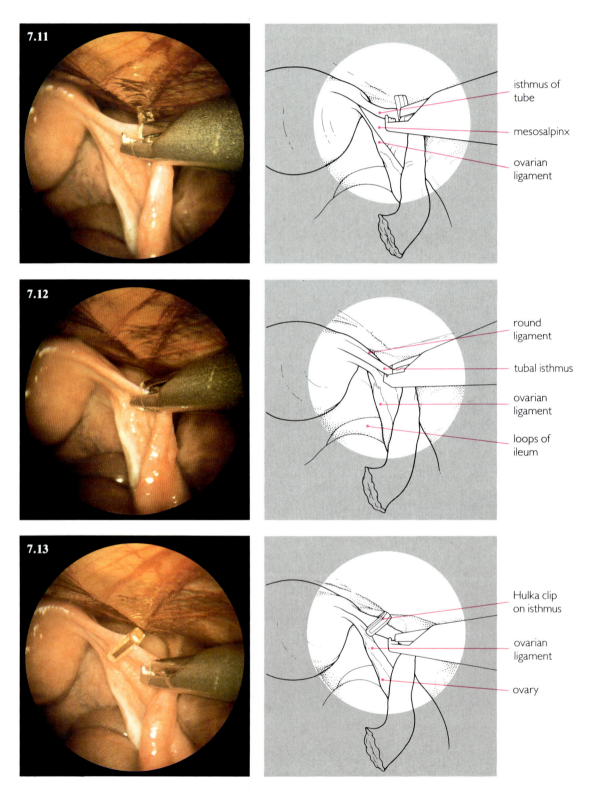

The Filshie clip has an outer frame of titanium with a silastic lining. Pressure on the curved upper jaw straightens and locks it under the hook on the lower jaw. The silastic lining expands as the tube is crushed and eventually transects the tube.

Application of the clip (Fig.7.14) is through a second suprapubic incision. A single hand movement locks the clip (Figs.7.15 & 7.16). The clips soon become peritonized and local tissue reaction is minimal. Adhesion of omentum or bowel to the clip is unusual.

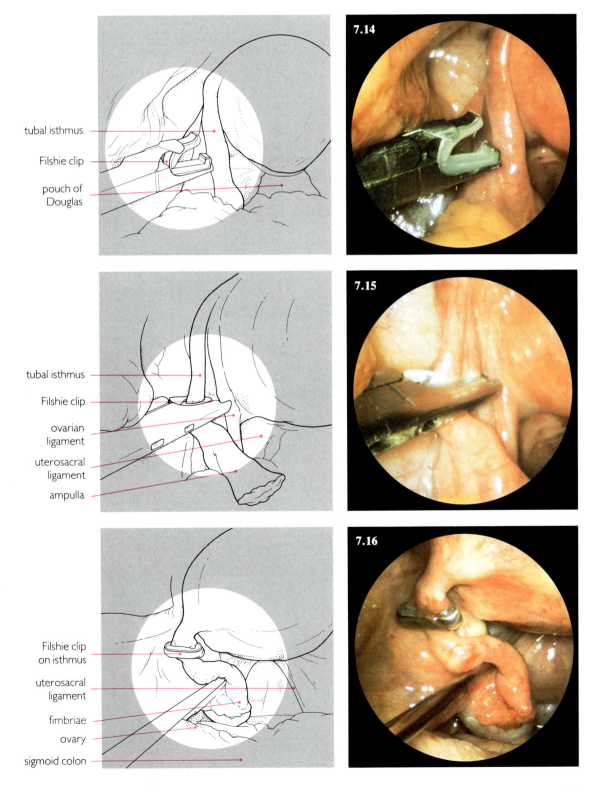

tubal isthmus

Filshie clip

pouch of Douglas

7.14

tubal isthmus

Filshie clip

ovarian ligament

uterosacral ligament

ampulla

7.15

Filshie clip on isthmus

uterosacral ligament

fimbriae

ovary

sigmoid colon

7.16

The Bleier (Fig.7.17) and Tupla (Fig.7.18) clips are alternative designs which work on the same principle; these are less commonly used than the other clips. In both, the mesosalpinx is penetrated by the locking mechanism, which can lead to bleeding.

The Yoon or Fallope ring is probably the most frequent method of female sterilization currently in use. Insertion is performed with either a single or double puncture technique. The former is quicker as only one incision is needed, but an operating laparoscope is required. Two rings can be loaded on the applicator at the same time, so that both tubes can be blocked with a single insertion of the instrument.

The Yoon ring is a silastic rubber band, 1mm in diameter, which is applied over a loop

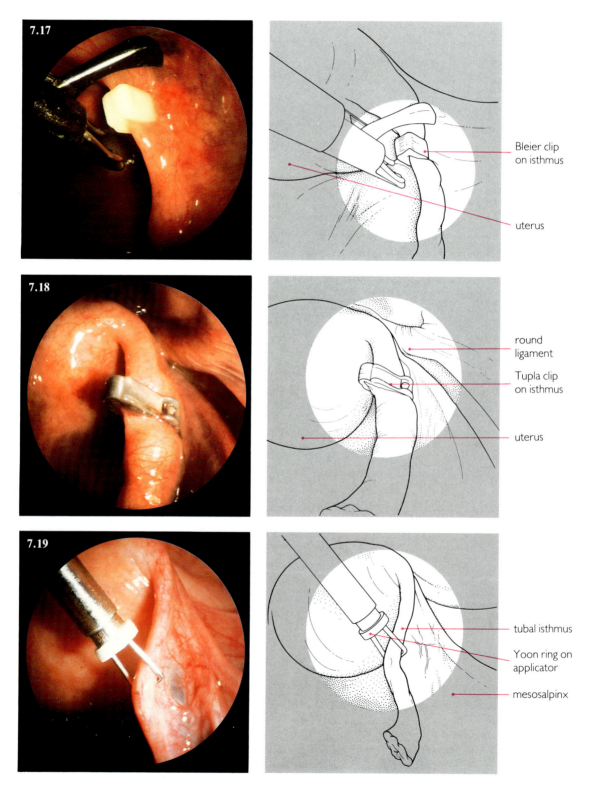

of tube. The full diameter of the tube is grasped with the applicator (Fig.7.19), a loop is formed by traction, and the applicator is advanced over the apex of the loop (Fig.7.20). The ring is then released (Fig.7.21) and the applicator withdrawn. The surgeon must be careful when drawing the loop up into the applicator, to avoid tearing the tube and causing bleeding from vessels in the mesosalpinx. This is more likely to happen if the tube is thickened or if its mobility is restricted by adhesions.

Complications

Complications due to clips are rare but salpingitis (Fig.7.22) occasionally occurs. Clip sterilization should be postponed if there is any evidence of infection at operation.

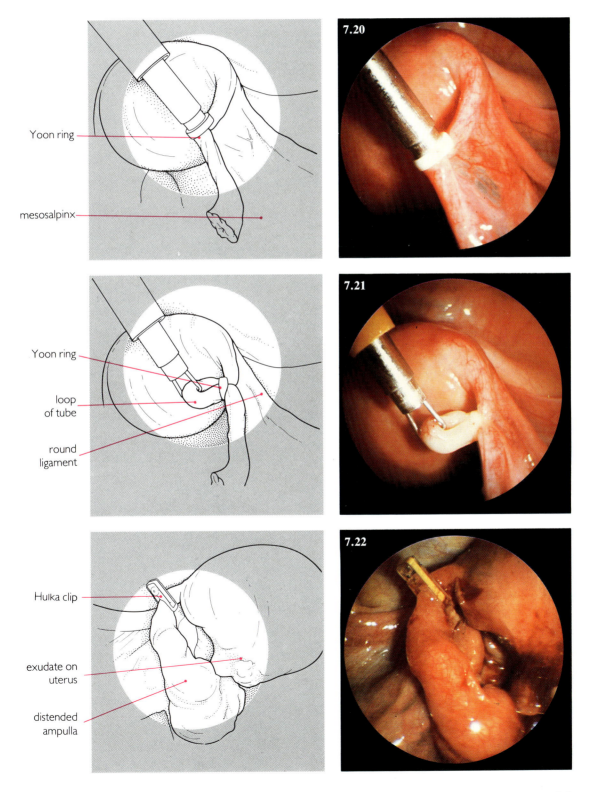

In theory, a tube which has been adequately blocked by clips, rings or electrocoagulation cannot recanalize. However, recanalization may occur after coagulation or cautery (Fig.7.23). A new channel can also form beyond the tip of a correctly applied clip (Fig.7.24).

This failure demonstrates that, even after a correctly performed sterilization, there remains a small, unavoidable risk of pregnancy. Failure of sterilization can also result from the whole thickness of the tube not being included in the loop (Fig.7.25).

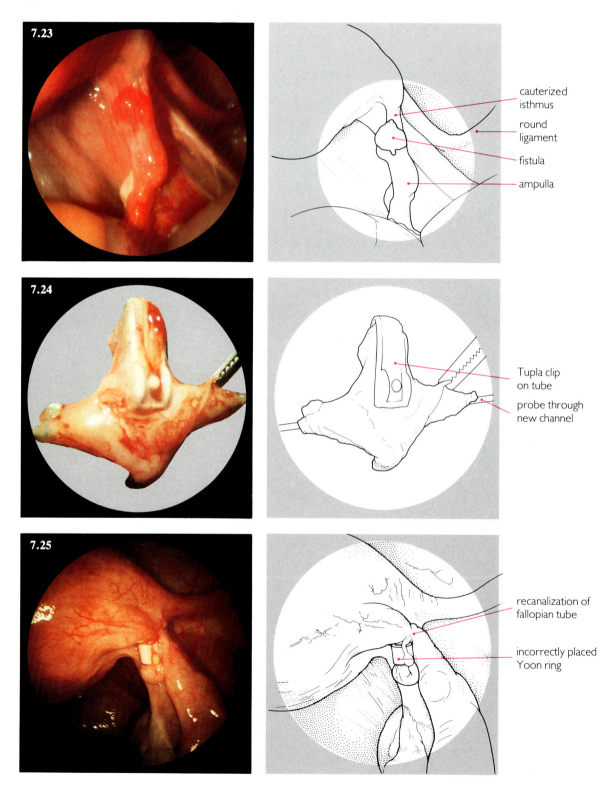

7.23

cauterized isthmus

round ligament

fistula

ampulla

7.24

Tupla clip on tube

probe through new channel

7.25

recanalization of fallopian tube

incorrectly placed Yoon ring

7.10

Ligation

Sterilization may also be achieved by laparoscopic ligation of the tube; a slip-knot is applied over a loop of isthmus, as in Pomeroy ligation. The slip-knot is based on the Roeder loop and is manufactured in both absorbable and non-absorbable sutures.

The tube is grasped with forceps and the Roeder loop passed over it (Figs.7.26 & 7.27). The noose is pulled tight (Fig.7.28) and the ligature cut. This method has the advantage that a segment of tube can be resected for histology. However, the operation involves a three-puncture technique to allow application of forceps, loop and scissors and is therefore not widely practised.

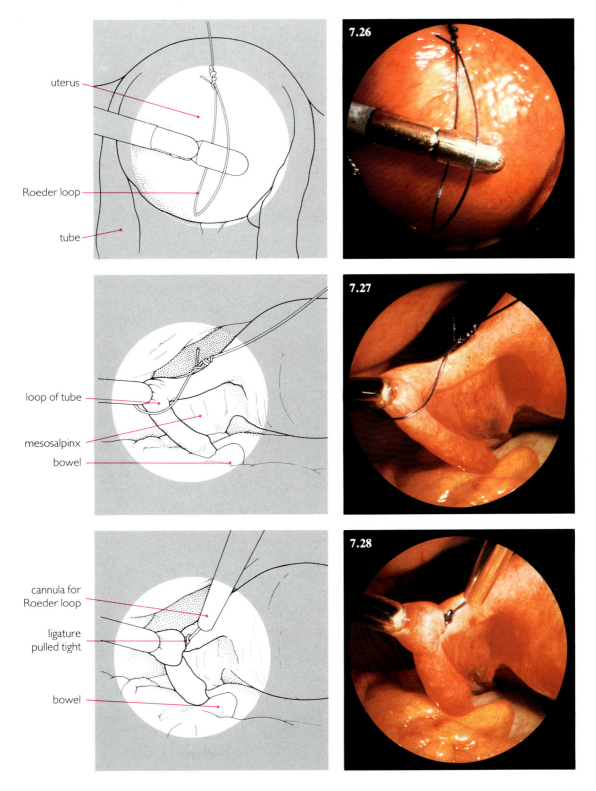

Hysteroscopic Sterilization

Trials are currently in progress to develop an effective method of hysteroscopic sterilization. Electrocautery, injection of chemicals and cryosurgery have all been tried but injection of occlusive substances and mechanical plugs appear to be the most promising. A plug is inserted into the tubal ostium via the operating channel of the hysteroscope using a clear plastic catheter. Methylene blue is injected and, if the tube is patent, this is followed by liquid silastic mixed with a catalyst (Fig.7.29). The silastic hardens in a few minutes and the catheter is removed, leaving the plug in the tube (Fig.7.30). Occasionally, some methylene blue leaks back into the uterus (Fig.7.31). The plug can be removed by pulling on the loop. At present, there is still doubt regarding both the efficiency of the sterilization and the success of reversal.

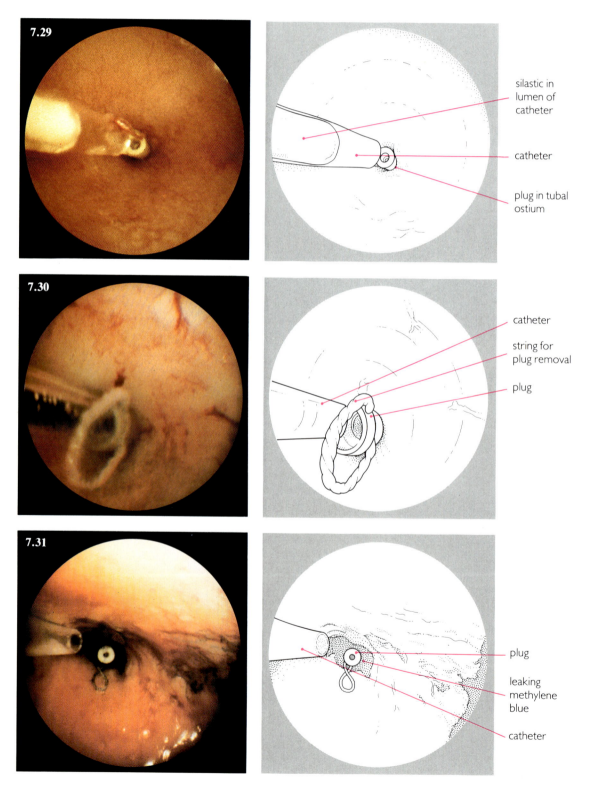

7.29 — silastic in lumen of catheter, catheter, plug in tubal ostium

7.30 — catheter, string for plug removal, plug

7.31 — plug, leaking methylene blue, catheter

8

PELVISCOPIC

SURGERY

The editors wish to acknowledge the contribution of
Professor Kurt Semm who provided all the endoscopic
photographs for this chapter.

Most gynaecologists use the laparoscope either to inspect the pelvic organs or to perform sterilization. The Kiel school, led by Semm, has developed operative laparoscopy, or pelviscopy, to an extent where they are able to substitute this form of surgery for laparotomy in a large number of cases.

Instruments for Pelviscopy

The first requirement for safe endoscopic surgery is the ability to control bleeding. Traditionally, unipolar or bipolar electro-coagulation has been used, but both produce an unnecessarily high temperature, with consequent risk of burning other organs. The Endocoagulator (Fig.8.1) uses a low-voltage current delivered at a temperature of 100–120°C for a period of time which is adequate to deliver heat to the jaws of the crocodile forceps (Fig.8.2). The dial records the operating temperature, and an audible signal informs the surgeon that the instrument is active without having to lift his eye from the operation field. The Endocoagulator is controlled by the surgeon using a foot pedal; the tone of the signal indicates when the temperature is dropping and coagulation is complete. Alternatively, heat can be applied to the distal end of the point coagulator to treat small bleeding vessels or to coagulate areas of endometriosis or the raw areas of the ovary after excision of a cyst.

8.1

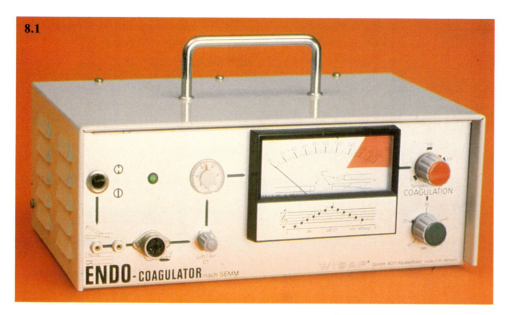

8.2

crocodile forceps

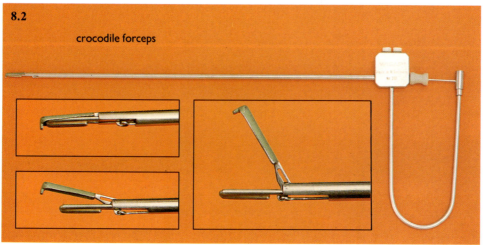

Control of intra-abdominal bleeding is achieved with the Roeder loop, or Ethibinder ligature (Fig.8.3), a slip-knot originally designed for tonsillectomy. The loop is passed down a 5mm cannula, the proximal end of the ligature applicator is snapped off, and the knot pushed downwards until the ligature is tight around the bleeding pedicle (Figs.8.4 & 8.5).

The Roeder loop is also available without a knot; it is passed around a band of tissue and drawn from the abdomen through the cannula before tying the knot. The loop is then tightened as before by pulling on the proximal end of the applicator. Larger vessels require additional ligatures to ensure haemostasis.

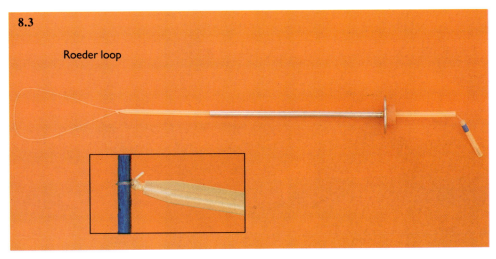

8.3

Roeder loop

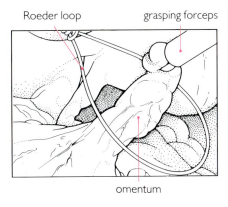

Roeder loop   grasping forceps

omentum

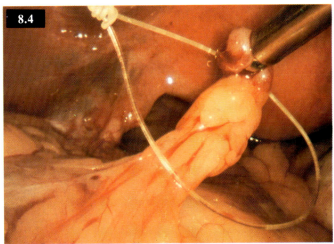

8.4

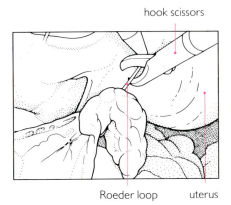

hook scissors

Roeder loop   uterus

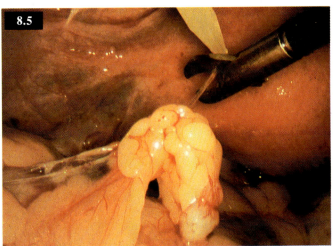

8.5

Incisions in the tube or ovary can be sutured, as in conventional surgery. A straight 4cm-long needle is introduced into the abdomen through a 5mm channel and grasped by needle-holding forceps. In Fig.8.6, the needle is being inserted into the cut edge of an ovary following resection of a cyst and is then pulled through with suture-tying forceps. A surgeon's knot is tied within the abdomen using both pairs of forceps (Figs.8.7 & 8.8). In addition to ovarian reconstruction following cyst excision, this technique can also be used for repair of the tube after pelviscopic reconstructive surgery or for insertion of a purse-string suture around the stump of the appendix after appendectomy.

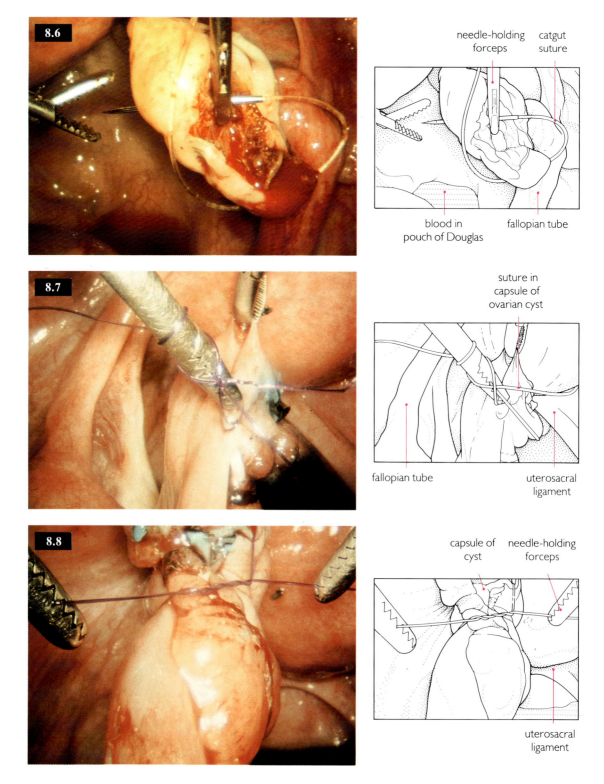

To complement these techniques, a new range of instruments has been designed to enable the surgeon to use both hands for operating through two or three channels. These instruments include atraumatic forceps (Fig.8.9) to hold the ovary or tube, grasping forceps for holding fibroids and cysts, and large scissors (Fig.8.10). While the surgeon is thus occupied, an assistant holds the laparoscope, using a teaching attachment or closed-circuit television to keep the operation site within his field of view.

An essential part of the procedure is removal of blood and debris during and after the operation. Ringer's solution is pumped through a 5mm irrigating cannula (Fig.8.11) from an Aquapurator pump or, more simply, from a 500ml plastic bottle with a pressure cuff; 1–3 litres of fluid is usually required to clear the pelvis.

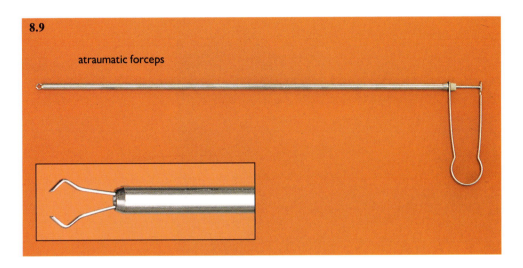

8.9 atraumatic forceps

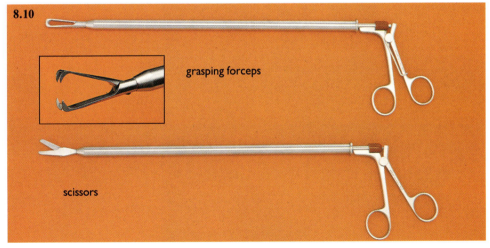

8.10 grasping forceps

scissors

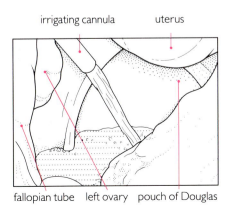

irrigating cannula   uterus

fallopian tube   left ovary   pouch of Douglas

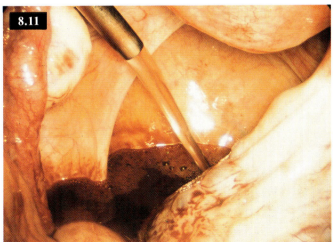

8.11

Adhesiolysis

The simplest pelviscopic operation is adhesiolysis, in which omental or peritoneal adhesions, which prevent inspection of the pelvis, are divided. These are often very fine and do not bleed when cut, especially if care is taken to find an avascular area. If necessary, however, they can be coagulated or ligated.

Atraumatic forceps and hook scissors are used to display and cut fine tubo-ovarian adhesions which restrict mobility of the tube (Figs.8.12 & 8.13). More extensive adhesions, which cover the ovary (Fig.8.14) and interfere with ovum release, and perifimbrial adhesions are dissected in the same way. These simple operative procedures are often sufficient to restore fertility without resorting to laparotomy.

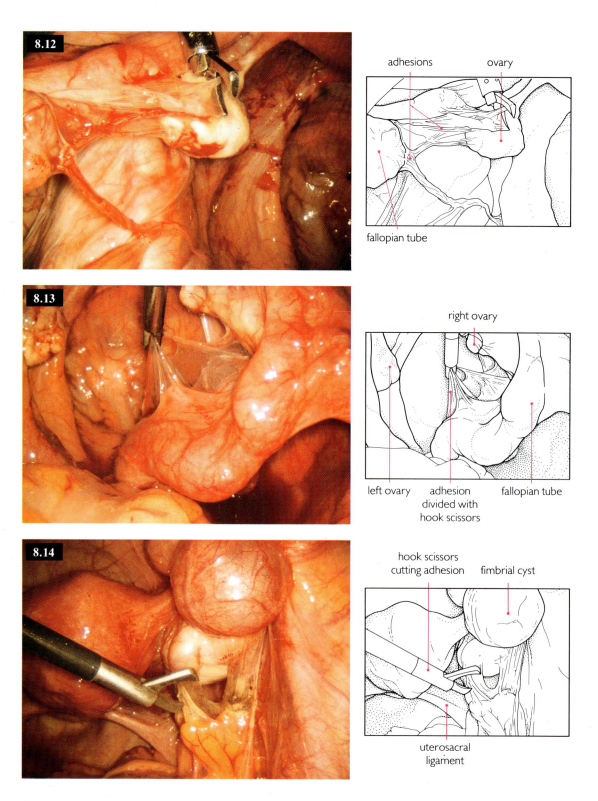

Ovariotomy

Luteal or follicular cysts are simply aspirated, but pathological cysts must be removed completely to avoid recurrence. The cyst is drained (Fig.8.15) and the fluid retained for cytological examination. The slack, empty capsule is held with forceps (Fig.8.16) while a ligature is placed around the redundant cyst wall, before removing it with scissors (Fig.8.17).

Sometimes, when the cyst has been aspirated and its capsule excised with scissors, a small part of it is left adhering to the ovary. This is easily peeled off with forceps, leaving a raw area on the ovary which is then either coagulated with the point coagulator or sutured. The pelvis is then washed out with Ringer's solution to remove blood and debris. This technique produces results similar to conventional laparotomy.

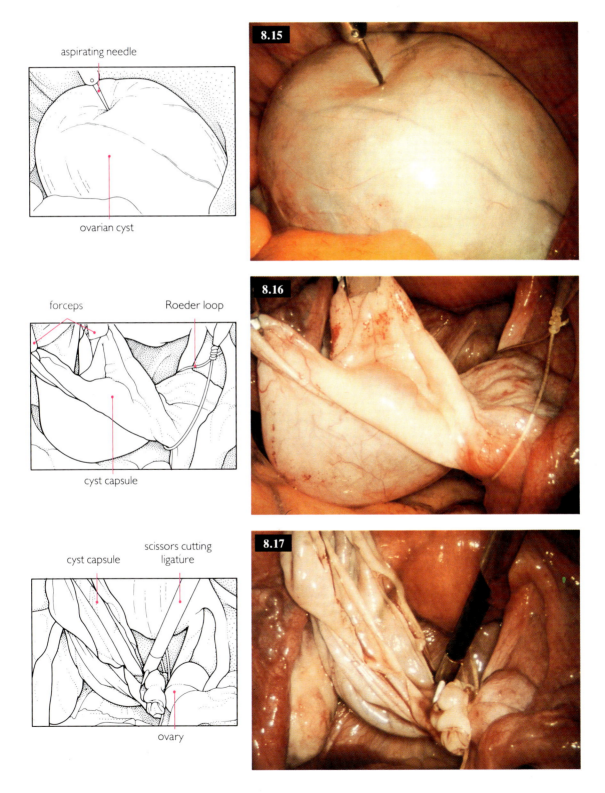

Oophorectomy

Pelviscopic oophorectomy can be used instead of laparotomy to treat oestrogen-dependent carcinoma of the breast; the former is less traumatic and has fewer complications.

Using large grasping forceps (Fig.8.18), the ovary is pulled towards the contralateral side of the pelvis to stretch and elongate the ovaricopelvic ligament. Three Roeder loops are placed around the ligament (Fig.8.19), which is then cut at right angles with scissors.

The stump is coagulated with the point coagulator (Fig.8.20) to ensure complete haemostasis and prevent formation of adhesions. The ovary is removed from the pelvis by grasping forceps, reducing its size by morcellement if necessary. The operation is completed by washing the pelvis with Ringer's solution and instillation of a hydrocortisone solution to prevent formation of further adhesions.

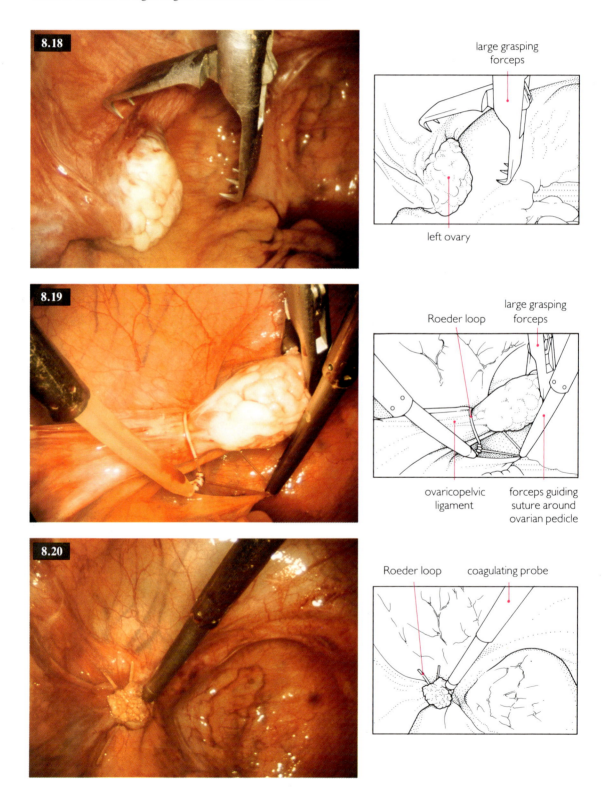

8.18

large grasping forceps

left ovary

8.19

Roeder loop

large grasping forceps

ovaricopelvic ligament

forceps guiding suture around ovarian pedicle

8.20

Roeder loop

coagulating probe

Myomectomy

When experience has been gained in simple adhesiolysis, the surgeon can progress to more advanced laparoscopic operations. These more complicated techniques can be taught with the help of closed-circuit television which allows all of the surgical team to see and assist the operation. Such operations include pelviscopic myomectomy and conservative tubal surgery.

Subserous fibroids (Fig.8.21) are held firmly with grasping forceps (Fig.8.22) and their pedicles coagulated with crocodile forceps (Fig.8.23). The pedicle is then divided with

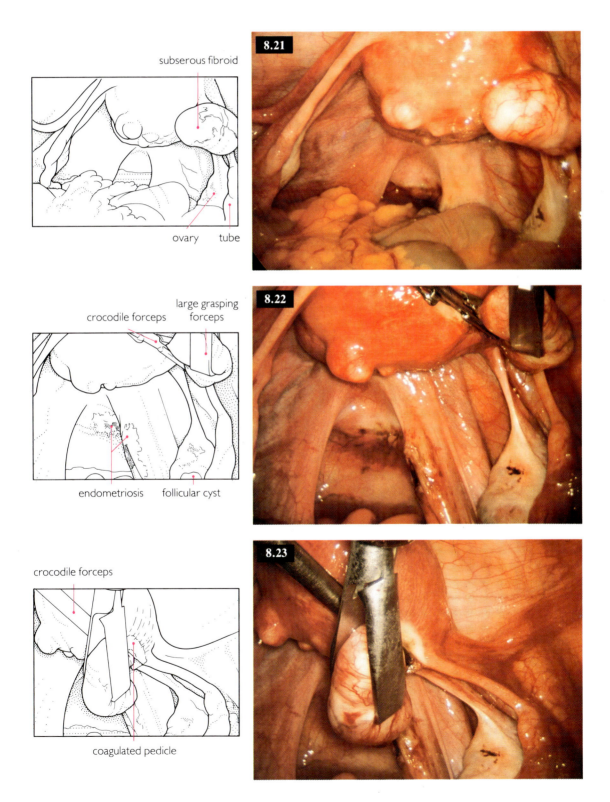

subserous fibroid

ovary   tube

large grasping forceps

crocodile forceps

endometriosis   follicular cyst

crocodile forceps

coagulated pedicle

scissors, freeing the fibroid from the uterus. The bed of the fibroid is coagulated again with the point coagulator (Fig.8.24) to ensure haemostasis. Fibroids close to the uterine cornua are best treated by laparotomy and microsurgery.

If, as in Fig. 8. 24, the fibroid is too large to be removed through the 10mm cannula, it is reduced by morcellement. This is achieved using either scissors or a tissue punch (Fig.8.25), which cuts the fibroid into small pieces, which can then be withdrawn through the lumen (Fig.8.26).

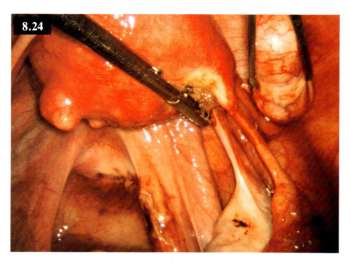

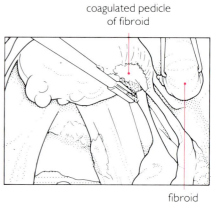

coagulated pedicle of fibroid

fibroid

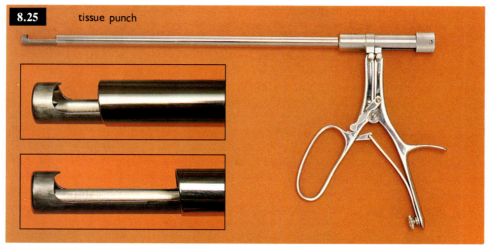

tissue punch

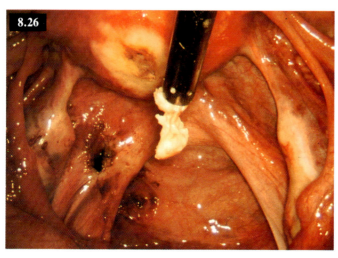

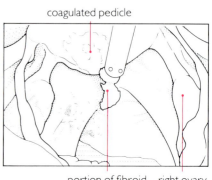

coagulated pedicle

portion of fibroid   right ovary

Ectopic pregnancy

Preliminary laparoscopy is necessary to confirm the diagnosis of tubal pregnancy. Conventional practice usually involves laparotomy with salpingectomy, although conservative surgery with preservation of the tube is becoming more widely accepted. However, a skilled laparoscopist can carry out salpingectomy if the tube is ruptured or, if the tube is still intact, remove the pregnancy and repair the tube.

The operation commences with peritoneal lavage (Fig.8.27) to remove blood and debris and give a clear view of the tube. If the tube is intact (Fig.8.28), the segment containing the pregnancy is coagulated and incised with hook scissors (Fig.8.29). The tube then retracts, the pregnancy sac extruding through the incision.

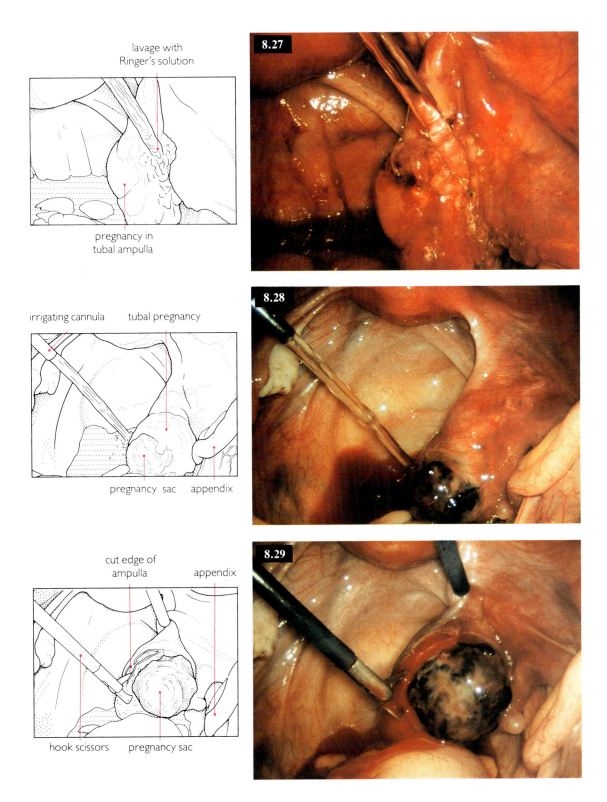

8.11

The cut edges are coagulated again if they bleed (Fig.8.30). Occasionally, the conceptus and blood clot must be removed piecemeal (Fig.8.31). Further lavage clears the pelvis of blood while the operation is in progress.

The incision in the tubal ampulla can be coagulated with the point coagulator to control bleeding, but this carries a risk of fistula formation. It is to better to suture the edges with an atraumatic stitch (Fig.8.32). Experience in Kiel and other European centres has shown that this procedure results in a high percentage of intrauterine pregnancies in patients whose contralateral tube has previously been removed.

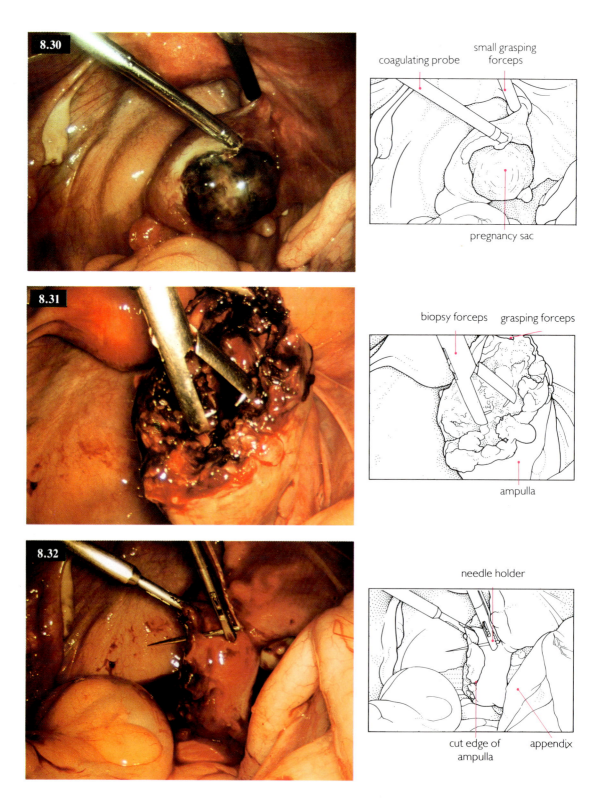

Salpingostomy

Microsurgery is necessary for treatment of cornual blockage and damage to the tubal isthmus, which may be caused by infection or operative sterilization. Distal blockage, however, can be treated with pelviscopic surgery.

The hydrosalpinx is distended with methylene blue injected through the cervix to confirm proximal patency and delineate the site of blockage. The tube is held by atraumatic forceps (Fig.8.33). The hydrosalpinx is opened with hook scissors (Fig.8.34), releasing methylene blue into the peritoneal cavity. The opening is enlarged with the ampulla dilator (Fig.8.35), which is inserted into the ampulla in the closed position and then opened and withdrawn. Gentle traction with forceps completes this stage of the operation.

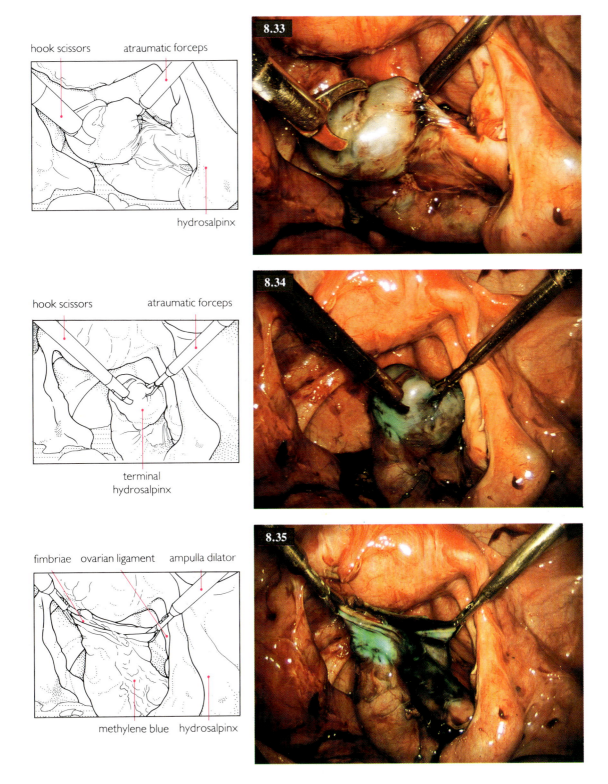

hook scissors   atraumatic forceps

hydrosalpinx

8.33

hook scissors   atraumatic forceps

terminal
hydrosalpinx

8.34

fimbriae   ovarian ligament   ampulla dilator

methylene blue   hydrosalpinx

8.35

A magnifying lens attached to the laparoscope magnifies the operation (x2) without limiting the field of vision, and allows the surgeon to confirm that the fimbriae are healthy (Fig.8.36) before completing the operation.

The edges of the opened hydrosalpinx are sutured to the peritoneum of the tube (Fig. 8.37) using a fine atraumatic nylon suture on a straight needle, which is tied with suture forceps (Fig.8.38).

Considerable technical expertise is required to perform this operation successfully, but the best results compare favourably with laparotomy and microsurgery. The main advantage of pelviscopic surgery is that ileus rarely occurs and thus the risk of adhesion formation is reduced.

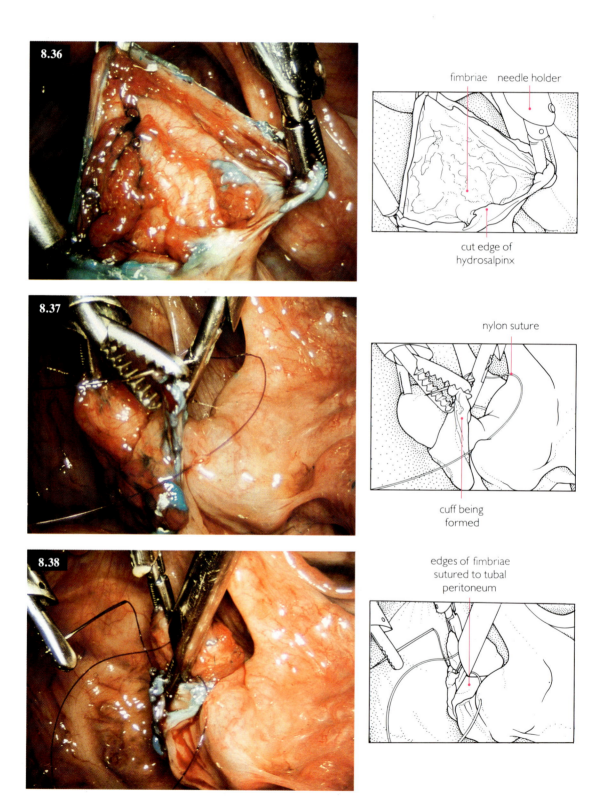

8.36

fimbriae   needle holder

cut edge of hydrosalpinx

8.37

nylon suture

cuff being formed

8.38

edges of fimbriae sutured to tubal peritoneum

9

HYSTEROSCOPY

Instruments for Hysteroscopy

Hysteroscopy is the examination of the uterine cavity using a fibreoptic endoscope and a proximal cold light source. The standard 4mm hysteroscope (Fig.9.1) gives a panoramic view of the cervical canal and uterine cavity and is sufficient for most diagnostic purposes.

The colpomicrohysteroscope (Fig.9.2) incorporates a facility to magnify from x1 to x150 to allow examination of the vascular and cellular structure of the endocervix and endo-metrium. When used at high magnification, the lens is in contact with the surface and complements colposcopy when the squamo-columnar junction is within the endocervical canal. Fine cellular detail can be observed after vital staining with Waterman's blue. An operating sheath (Fig.9.3), which allows scissors, diathermy probes and biopsy forceps to be introduced for intrauterine surgery under direct vision, is optional.

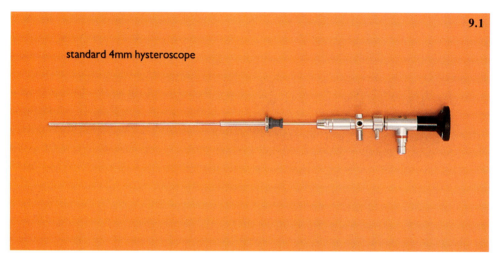

9.1

standard 4mm hysteroscope

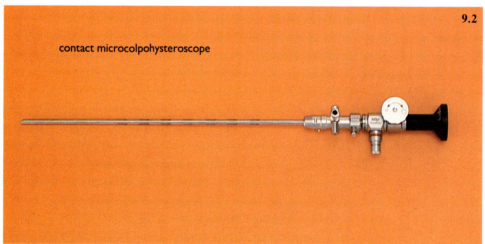

9.2

contact microcolpohysteroscope

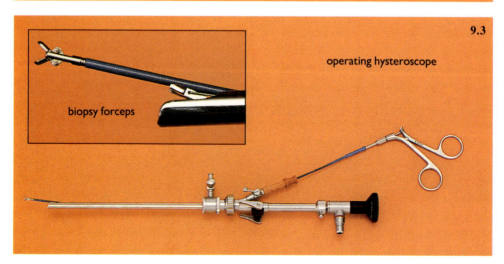

9.3

operating hysteroscope

biopsy forceps

Since the uterine cavity must be distended to obtain a clear view, the hysteroscope incorporates a sheath through which gas or fluid passes from the tip. Carbon dioxide is delivered from a Hysteroflator or Metromat (Fig.9.4) at a flow rate of not more than 100ml/min under low pressure. Leakage of gas around the cervix may be prevented by a vacuum cup (Fig.9.5), but usually the pressure exerted by the cervix on the hysteroscope is sufficient. Only a small quantity of carbon dioxide enters the peritoneal cavity through the fallopian tubes and this is readily absorbed. The pneumoperitoneum apparatus for laparoscopy must not be used for hysteroscopy because the high pressure and flow rate are dangerous.

If fluid is used to distend the uterine cavity, a solution of 5% dextrose washes away any blood and allows a satisfactory view of all stages of the menstrual cycle. Alternatively, Hyscon (32% dextrose) coalesces the blood into globules while the medium remains clear. Normally, about 10ml of Hyscon is needed. The instruments must be carefully washed after use because the fluid is highly viscous and may block their moving parts.

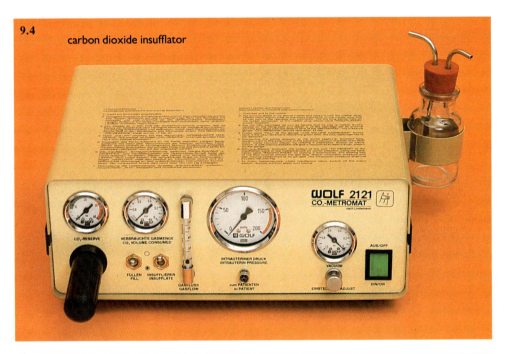

9.4 carbon dioxide insufflator

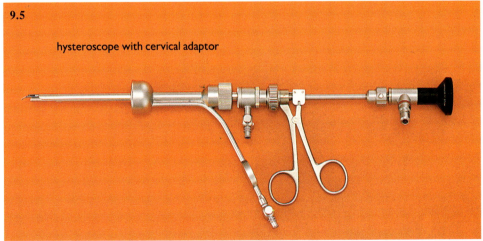

9.5

hysteroscope with cervical adaptor

Normal Hysteroscopic Findings

Hysteroscopy can be carried out under a light general anaesthetic or, as an outpatient procedure, with paracervical block. If the internal os is sufficiently dilated, no anaesthetic is required as gentle distention of the uterus is painless.

The hysteroscope is introduced through the external os and is slowly advanced along the cervical canal. The normal canal appears smooth on panoramic view, but when magnified x20 (Fig.9.6), the folds of the columnar epithelium and the openings of the endocervical glands are seen. As the telescope approaches the internal os, the cavity comes into view (Fig.9.7).

The fundus (Fig.9.8) appears saddle-shaped with a cornual orifice on each side. The colour of the normal endometrium varies with the menstrual cycle from the pallor of the post-menstrual, to the redness of the vascular pre-menstrual phase. Similarly, the postmeno-pausal endometrium is thin and avascular.

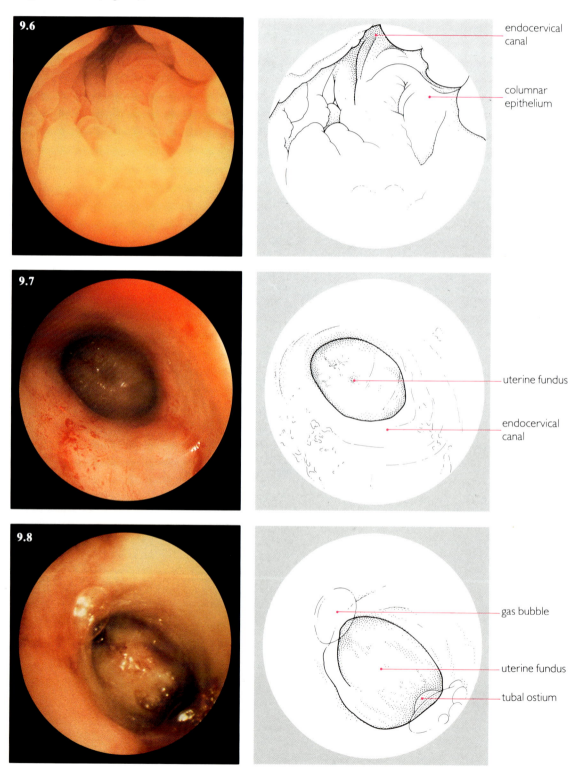

9.6 — endocervical canal / columnar epithelium

9.7 — uterine fundus / endocervical canal

9.8 — gas bubble / uterine fundus / tubal ostium

As the telescope approaches the fundus, the light intensity increases. Rotation and angling of the telescope brings the tubal ostia into view. When the telescope is almost in contact with the endometrium, the ostium nearly fills the field of vision. Further magnification allows the proximal 1–2 mm of the intramural portion of the tube to be inspected (Fig.9.9).

When the ostia are observed over a short period of time, they are seen to open and close as gas escapes through the tube into the peritoneal cavity (Figs.9.10 & 9.11). This is a normal physiological finding: failure to appreciate this at hysterosalpingography or hydropertubation may lead to misdiagnosis of cornual blockage.

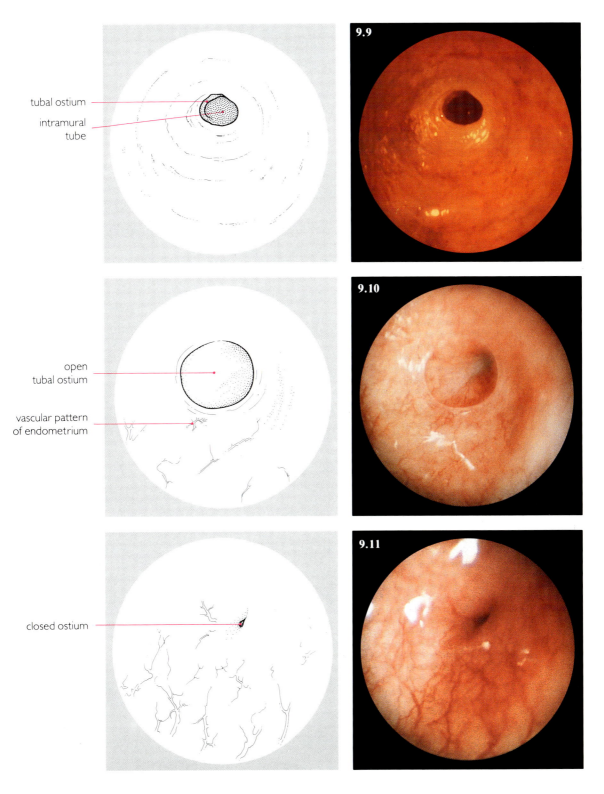

tubal ostium
intramural tube

open tubal ostium

vascular pattern of endometrium

closed ostium

Tumours

Benign endometrial polyps are distinguishable from carcinoma by their appearance. They are smooth, discrete, shiny and quite often vascular (Fig.9.12). It is difficult to differentiate adenomatous mucous polyps by appearance alone, and so biopsy and histological confirmation are required. Bleeding following biopsy or curettage may obscure vision when gas insufflation is used, but if dextrose is the distending medium, the blood will be washed away by continuous irrigation.

A benign mucous polyp (Fig.9.13) may be so large as to distort the uterine cavity, but shows no signs of necrosis or ulceration. The polyps may be multiple, each with a discrete outline (Fig.9.14), but together they may cause considerable irregularity of the uterine cavity.

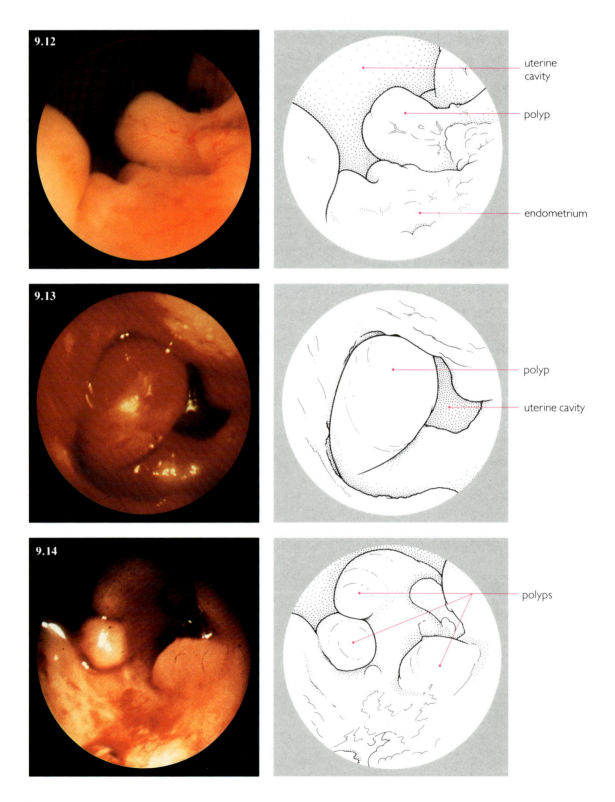

In patients with secondary dysmenorrhoea and menorrhagia, hysteroscopy is especially valuable for detecting small submucous fibroids. The appearance is characteristic: the fibroid is smooth and paler in colour than the rest of the endometrium (Fig.9.15) because it is less vascular. Hysteroscopy is more accurate than hysterography because in the latter, air bubbles cause artefacts and it is also impossible to differentiate a fibroid from an endometrial polyp by this method. If the submucous fibroid is small and has a narrow pedicle (Fig.9.16), it can be removed under direct vision. More usually, however, it is intramural, becoming submucous, and the fibroid can then only be removed by laparotomy.

In those who develop menorrhagia due to an intrauterine device, hysteroscopy may help to exclude other pathology (Fig.9.17).

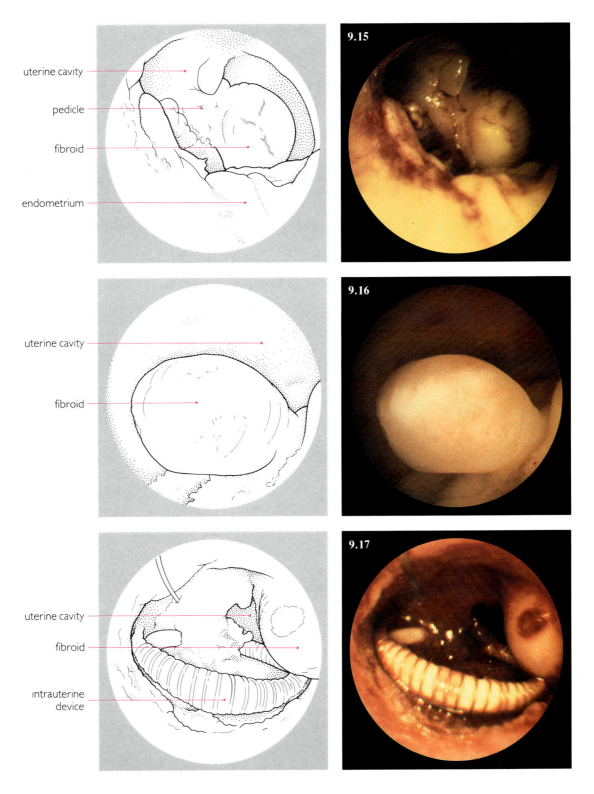

Hysteroscopy is not usually performed in patients with postmenopausal bleeding to diagnose carcinoma of the endometrium. However, there are advantages in assessing the size of the tumour and detecting extension into the cervical canal. There is a theoretical risk of spilling malignant cells into the peritoneum which, although not confirmed by clinical experience, has not been completely disproved. An endometrial carcinoma (Fig. 9.18) is irregular in outline and vascular in pattern, and the surface may ulcerate and bleed (Fig.9.19). Tumours of this size will be detected by curettage but a small discrete tumour could be missed, as in Fig.9.20, where there is also a small submucous fibroid.

Tubal Catheterization

When investigating infertility, the cornu can be catheterized to confirm patency of the intra-

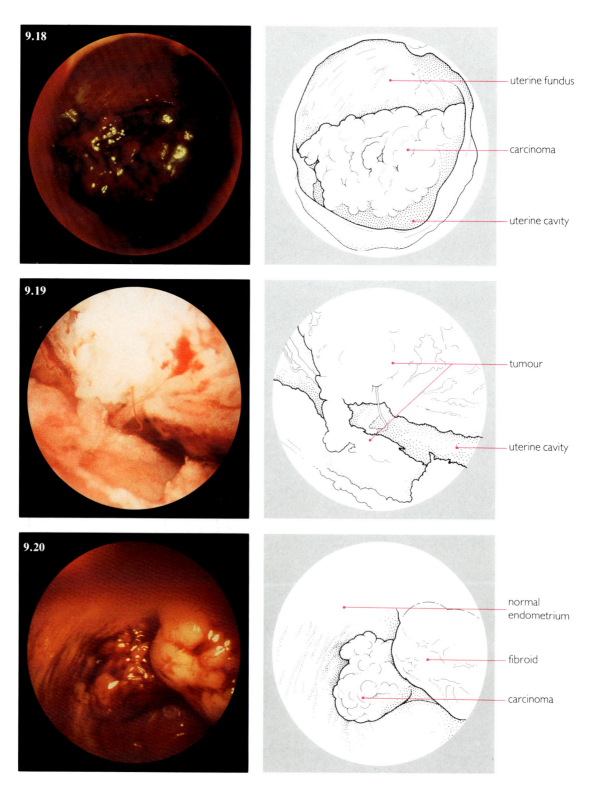

mural portion of the tube (Fig.9.21). Using an operating hysteroscope, a flexible nylon catheter, 1mm in diameter, is inserted through the cornual ostium into the intramural portion of the tube (Fig.9.22); A very fine catheter will reach the isthmus (Fig.9.23), but there is a danger of damage to, or even perforation of the endosalpinx. The use of tubal catheterization for injecting sclerosing fluids or plugs for sterilization is currently undergoing clinical trials. It has been suggested that intra-tubal artificial insemination may be of value in severe oligospermia, and this is also a possible route for gamete intrafallopian transfer (GIFT).

True cornual blockage is usually caused by fibrosis of the whole length of the intramural tube, secondary to infection. Occasionally, there is a thin occluding membrane which the catheter will pierce.

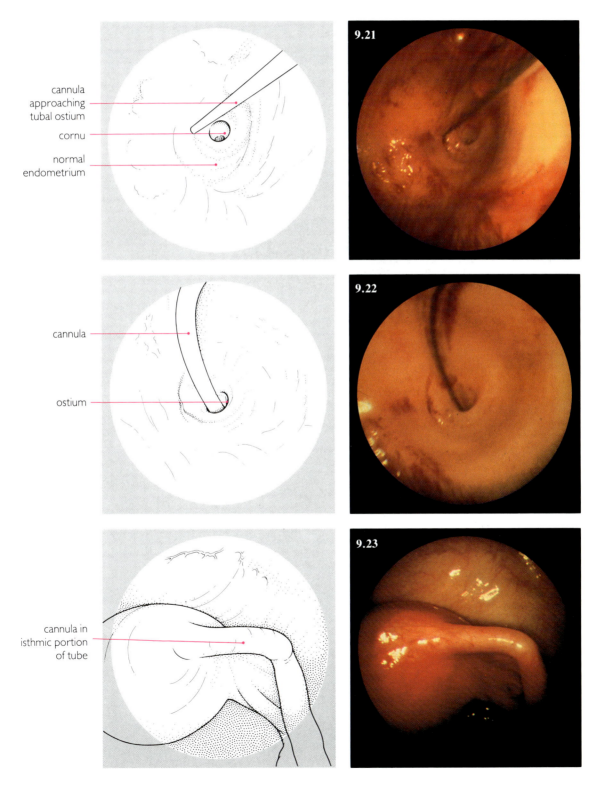

9.21

cannula approaching tubal ostium

cornu

normal endometrium

9.22

cannula

ostium

9.23

cannula in isthmic portion of tube

Intrauterine Devices

An intrauterine device which cannot be removed is a common gynaecological problem. Even if the thread protrudes from the cervix, removal may be difficult because the coil is partly embedded in the uterine wall (Fig.9.24). If the thread is not visible, the coil is either lying in the uterine cavity or has perforated the uterus. Ultrasound will usually locate the device in the cavity, but removal can be difficult. Hysteroscopy allows both the position and type of the coil to be seen (Fig.9.25) and it can then be removed by grasping forceps.

Hysteroscopy can also be of value in pregnancy to define the position of the sac, especially with a missed abortion (Fig.9.26); it also allows removal of a coil without disturbing a viable pregnancy.

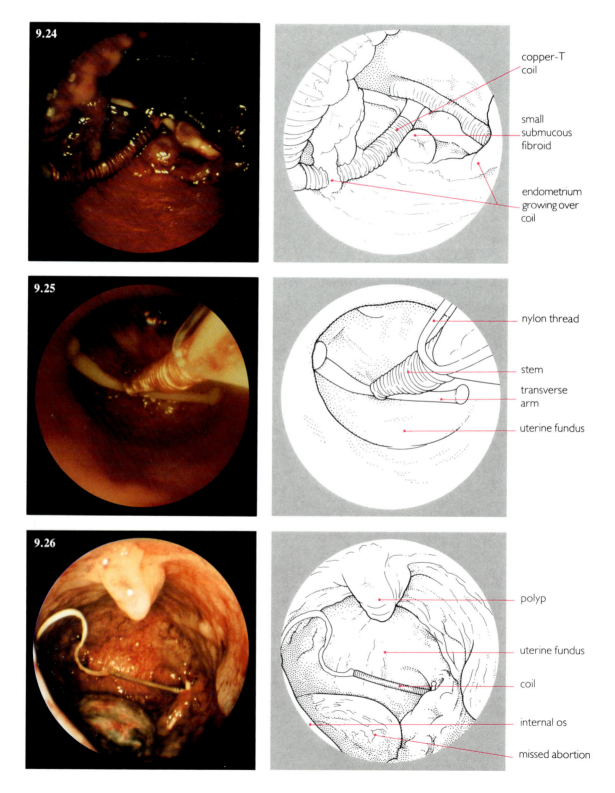

9.24 — copper-T coil, small submucous fibroid, endometrium growing over coil

9.25 — nylon thread, stem, transverse arm, uterine fundus

9.26 — polyp, uterine fundus, coil, internal os, missed abortion

Pregnancy Related Conditions

Bleeding following evacuation of the uterus is usually due to retained products of conception; this can be confirmed by hysteroscopy (Fig.9.27). Vigorous curettage in the puerperal or postabortal uterus, or subclinical sepsis may lead to uterine synechiae. The patient presents with oligomenorrhoea or secondary amenorrhoea. Minor degrees are asymptomatic, but they may be associated with infertility or recurrent abortion.

The synechiae range from relatively fine strands (Fig.9.28) to thick bands of tissue which may almost divide the uterus into two separate cavities; this must be differentiated from a bicornuate uterus (Fig.9.29). The synechiae can be divided with scissors, following which menstruation returns to normal. A coil inserted for two cycles should prevent their reforming.

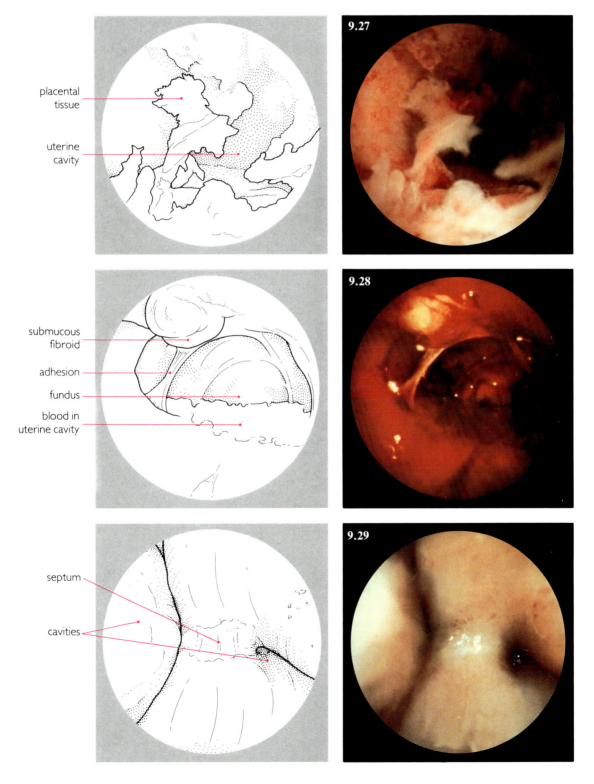

Laser Ablation of Endometrium

During menstruation, the endometrium peels away from the uterine wall (Fig.9.30), beginning at the fundus. In cases of severe menorrhagia, most patients are offered hysterectomy, but if this is contraindicated or declined, or if drug therapy fails, hysteroscopic laser vaporization of the endometrium (Goldrath, 1985) is an alternative treatment which is currently under clinical trial.

Preliminary hysteroscopy and curettage is performed to exclude malignancy, polyps and myomata, and the endometrium is rendered atrophic with danazol, 800mg/d for three weeks. Using Nd:YAG laser transmitted along a quartz fibreoptic rod, and 5% dextrose in saline as the distending medium, the endometrium is partially destroyed under hysteroscopic control. A large volume of fluid is

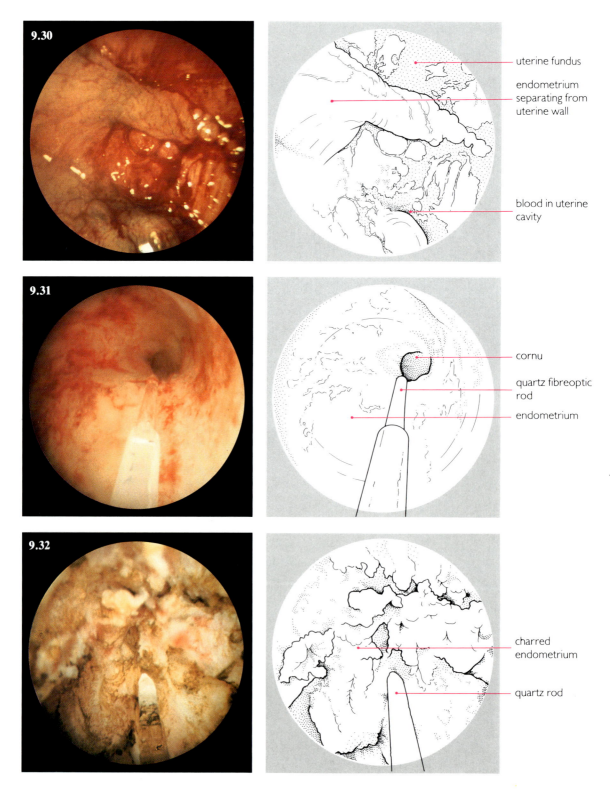

9.30 — uterine fundus / endometrium separating from uterine wall / blood in uterine cavity

9.31 — cornu / quartz fibreoptic rod / endometrium

9.32 — charred endometrium / quartz rod

required to keep the field of vision clear, most of it escaping through the cervix and past the telescope. In addition, some fluid escapes into the peritoneal cavity and is absorbed into the circulation, where it may cause cardiovascular overloading, which quickly responds to diuretic therapy.

The endometrium is treated systematically from fundus to cervix under constant visual control. Laser is first applied to the uterine cornua (Fig.9.31), followed by the fundal endometrium, which appears blackened when vaporized (Figs.9.32 & 9.33). Islands of untreated tissue (Fig.9.34) are dealt with as they are discovered. The end result is a charred endometrium (Fig.9.35) with intrauterine adhesions, resulting in amenorrhoea or oligomenorrhoea and infertility. In Goldrath's series, only 9 out of 260 patients eventually required hysterectomy.

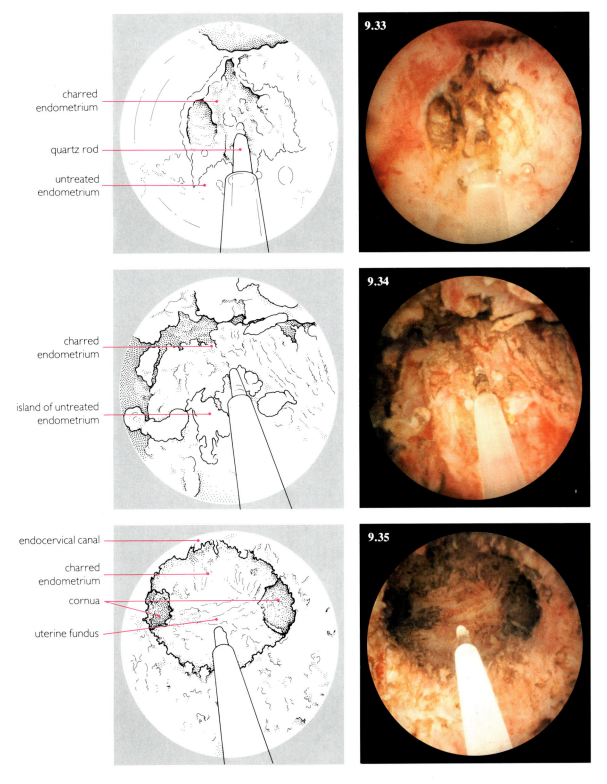

Microhysteroscopy

The squamous cells of the endocervix or the columnar epithelium of the endometrium can be examined with the colpomicrohysteroscope. This is especially valuable when the transformation zone lies within the endocervix. Staining with Lugol's iodine and Waterman's blue differentiates the squamous from the columnar epithelium with gland openings (Fig.9.36). At a higher magnification, the cellular pattern of the cervical canal is seen (Fig.9.37).

Reference

Goldrath MH (1986). In *Gynaecological Laser Surgery*. Edited by F Sharp & J A Jordan. pp 253-265. New York: Perinatology Press.

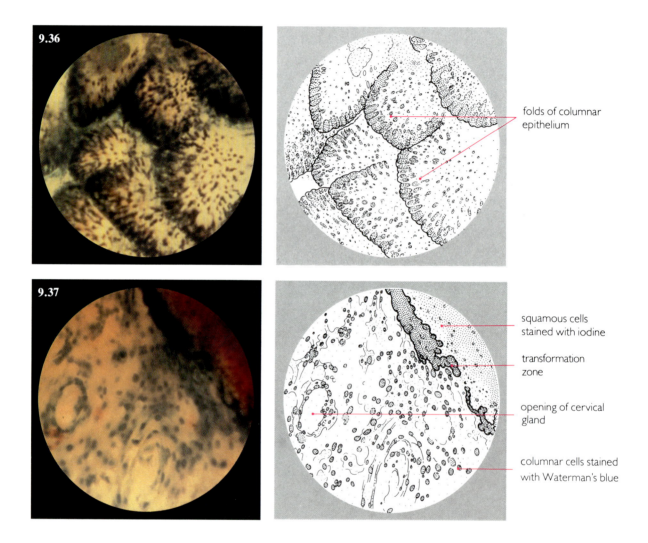

folds of columnar epithelium

squamous cells stained with iodine

transformation zone

opening of cervical gland

columnar cells stained with Waterman's blue

SALPINGOSCOPY

I. A.   BROSENS
with the technical assistance of
L. de Simpelaere

Direct visualization of the fallopian tube allows study of the tubal mucosa in subfertile patients. Mucosal lesions such as flattening or adhesions of the folds, erosions, polyps, loss of cilia and occlusion have all been described in tubal infertility. Studies of hydrosalpinges carried out in Leuven have shown a high correlation between the appearance of the tube and subsequent pregnancy.

Salpingoscopy at laparotomy
Salpingoscopy was originally performed during laparotomy for tubal reconstructive surgery; the presence or absence of mucosal pathology was used as a prognostic index. A Hamou hysteroscope in a 5.2mm diameter sheath is introduced through the fimbriae and connected to a saline infusion set which is run at a moderately fast rate to distend the tubal lumen. This allows the hysteroscope to be inserted into the tube as far as the ampulloisthmic junction.

When the telescope enters the tube, normal fimbriae are visible, with several major and minor folds leading towards the infundibulum (Fig. 10.1). As the telescope is advanced into

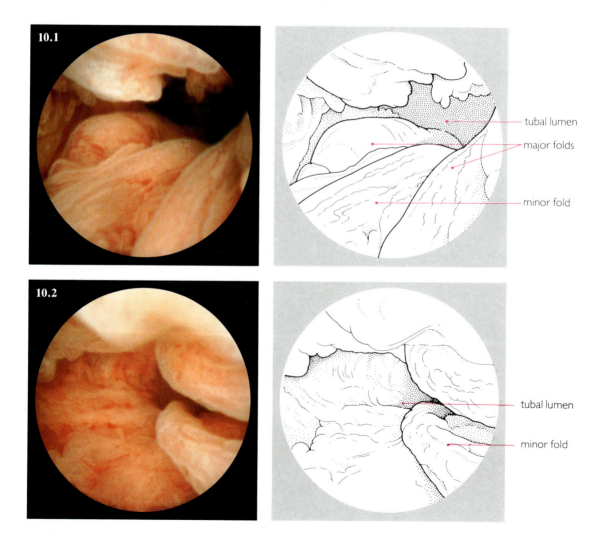

tubal lumen

major folds

minor fold

tubal lumen

minor fold

the ampulla, similar major and minor folds are seen but when the ampulloisthmic junction is reached, the major folds are replaced by minor folds (Fig. 10.2). If methylene blue is injected through the cervix, the folds are stained blue (Fig. 10.3). In Fig. 10.4, three major folds in the ampulla are seen bulging into the lumen.

The Hamou colpomicrohysteroscope allows the endosalpinx to be magnified and permits the microvascular structure of the major folds to be studied in detail (Fig. 10.5).

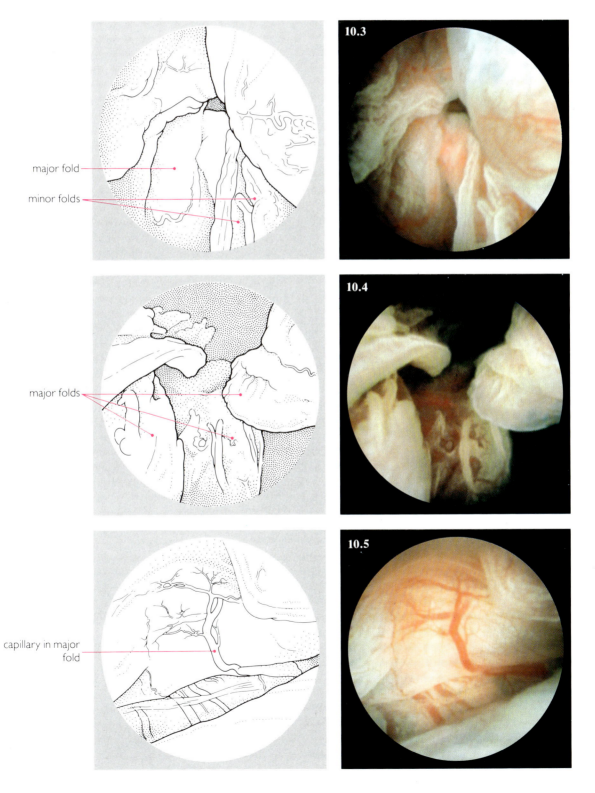

Salpingoscopy at laparoscopy

An alternative method of salpingoscopy has been developed, in which a rigid 3mm telescope is passed along the channel of an operating laparoscope. The essential part of the operation is the alignment of the fallopian tube with the axis of the laparoscope; this can be achieved by manipulating the uterus with a cervical cannula. By rotating the uterus and presenting the adnexa on its anterior surface, the fimbriae and ampulla become easily accessible, although sometimes the tube needs to be held steady and aligned with atraumatic forceps, which are introduced through a second incision (Fig. 10.6). If necessary, peritubal adhesions are divided laparoscopically to mobilize the tube. A probe is used to identify the abdominal ostium and the salpingoscope is introduced with its sheath connected to a saline infusion set. Using a moderately fast flow rate the tube is distended, allowing the telescope to be advanced under

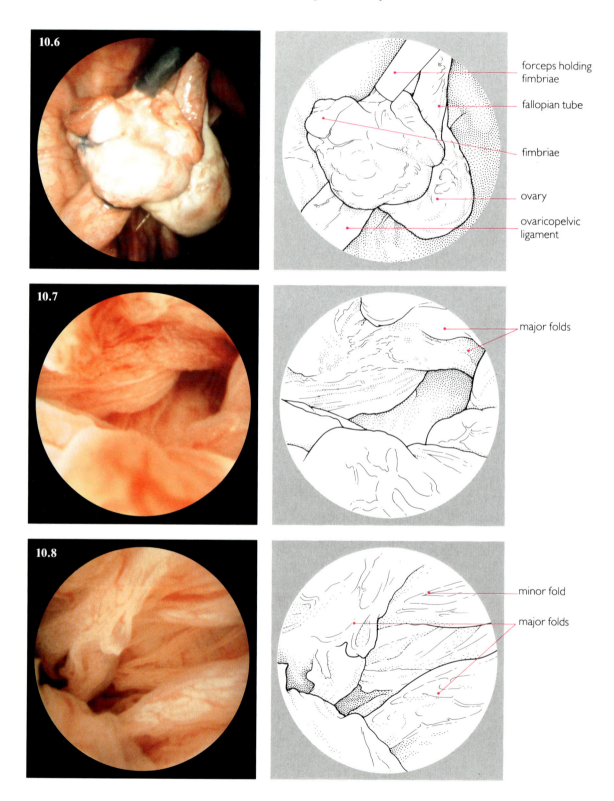

direct vision. Fig. 10.7 shows the laparoscopic view of the normal fold pattern of the infundibulum, while Fig. 10.8 shows the major and minor folds of the ampulla.

If hydrosalpinx is discovered at laparoscopy, further investigation by salpingoscopy will help to assess the potential value of tubal microsurgery. If the endosalpinx can be inspected, a decision on the prognosis can be made without subjecting the patient to laparotomy. First, the hydrosalpinx must be mobilized with scissor dissection; haemostasis is achieved with endocoagulation, and the terminal end is brought into line with the laparoscope (Fig. 10.9). Holding the infundibulum with atraumatic forceps, the tube is incised with hook scissors, allowing the methylene blue injected through the cervix to spill out, and thus demonstrate proximal tubal patency (Fig. 10.10). The salpingoscope can now be introduced and the lumen inspected. A tube which is distended but in which the major and minor folds are preserved (Fig. 10.11) indicates a good prognosis.

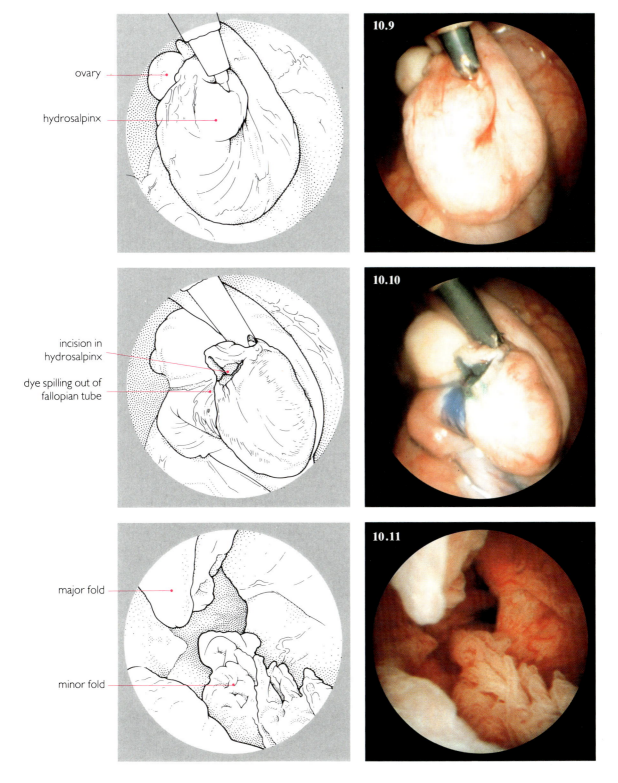

ovary

hydrosalpinx

10.9

incision in hydrosalpinx

dye spilling out of fallopian tube

10.10

major fold

minor fold

10.11

In more marked degrees of hydrosalpinx, the folds in the infundibulum may be preserved, but may appear more widely separated from each other than normal (Fig. 10.12), which supports the diagnosis of tubal damage. In a more serious case, the major tubal folds in the ampulla are flattened (Fig. 10.13) and the tube appears thin-walled and atrophic.

In addition to flattening of the folds and widening of the space between them, adhesions are also occasionally seen (Fig. 10. 14); this is always of poor prognostic significance. A woman presenting with these signs has little chance of achieving a pregnancy following tubal microsurgery and consideration should be given to in vitro fertilization.

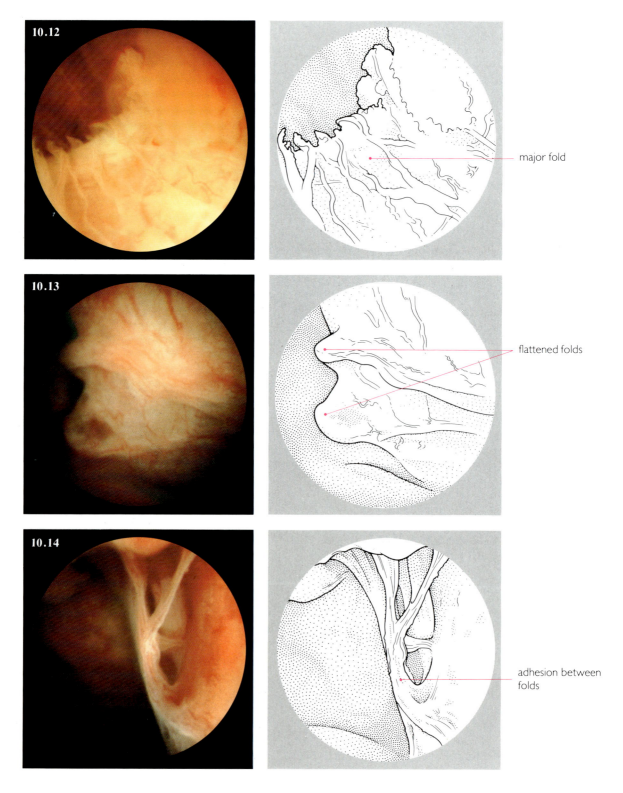

10.12

major fold

10.13

flattened folds

10.14

adhesion between folds

In hydrosalpinx with extensive tubal destruction, the fold pattern disappears and thick, firm adhesions form in the ampulla (Fig. 10.15). This situation is hopeless and the woman will not conceive spontaneously.

Rarely, a pseudohydrosalpinx or tubal herniation is found. The underlying pathology is probably aplasia of the myosalpinx, pro-ducing herniation of the mucosa. Examination of the infundibulum shows a normal fold pattern (Fig. 10.16), but when the telescope is advanced into the ampulla, the lumen of the tube is seen to be grossly distended and the wall thin and transparent (Fig. 10.17). The major folds are absent in the distended segment; minor folds are present but are flattened.

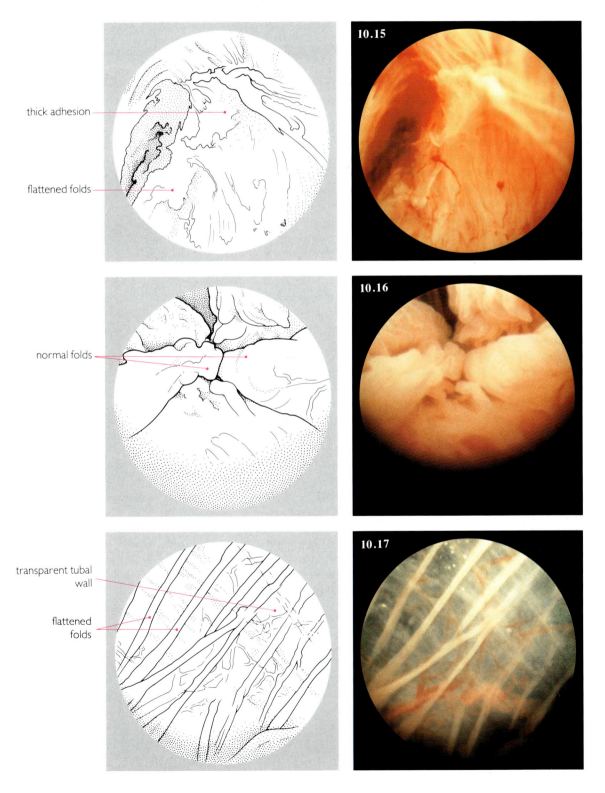

thick adhesion

flattened folds

10.15

normal folds

10.16

transparent tubal wall

flattened folds

10.17

Flexible salpingoscopy

Recently, 3mm flexible endoscopes, which are fine enough to be passed into the fallopian tube and directed through the tortuous endosalpinx, have been produced; this has allowed the development of flexible salpingoscopy. The telescope is introduced through an operating laparoscope and advanced along the tube under direct vision (Fig. 10.18), using fine tuning of the controls and rotary finger movements to guide it. The field of vision is not as wide as with a rigid telescope and the pattern of the fibreoptic bundles is visible, but adhesions between the fimbriae (Fig. 10.19) are easily seen. As with the rigid salpingoscope, the flexible telescope can be used to assess the result of tubal surgery for hydrosalpinx, as in Fig. 10.20 where the flattening of the folds indicates irreparable tubal damage.

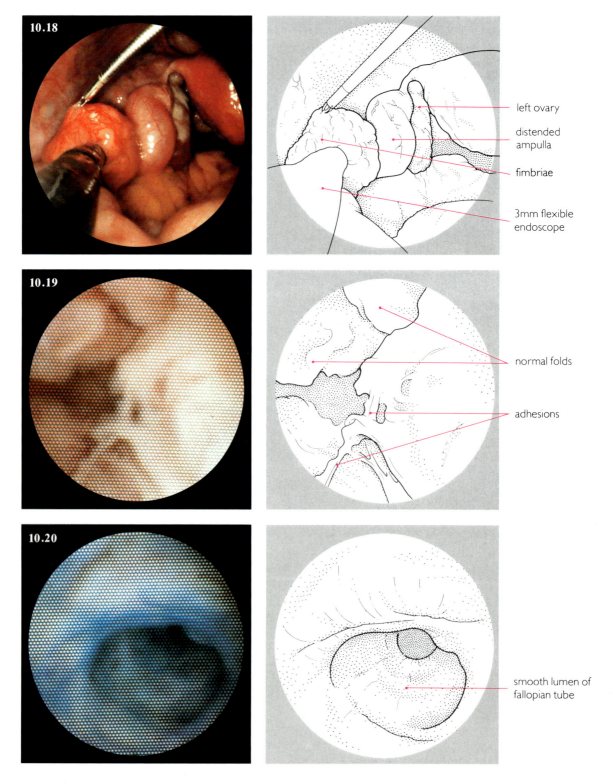

10.18

- left ovary
- distended ampulla
- fimbriae
- 3mm flexible endoscope

10.19

- normal folds
- adhesions

10.20

- smooth lumen of fallopian tube

CULDOSCOPY

J. S. SCOTT

K. W. HANCOCK

Culdoscopy provides a safe and effective method of visualizing the female pelvic organs by inserting a peritoneoscope through the posterior vaginal fornix into the pouch of Douglas or cul-de-sac. The procedure was introduced in the early 1940s but was replaced by laparoscopy in many centres in the 1960s, when fibreoptic lighting systems were developed. This form of illumination is now also standard for culdoscopy and therefore this approach has continued to be used in a number of centres throughout the world.

Technique

Culdoscopy has several advantages over laparoscopy. There is no need to induce a pressure pneumoperitoneum, it avoids the risk of damage to bowel which may be adherent to the anterior abdominal wall as a result of previous surgery, and only two thin layers of tissue, the posterior vaginal wall and the pouch of Douglas peritoneum, need to be pierced, allowing a more gentle puncture without a trocar to be employed. Even in obese patients the tissue thickness is only 2mm. Culdoscopy is contraindicated if the pouch of Douglas has adhesions which can be detected on bimanual examination. In experienced hands, the complications of this procedure are few and none are serious.

The patient is usually given general anaesthesia with endotracheal intubation. Bimanual examination is performed to ensure that the fingers can meet behind the uterus, thus excluding adhesions. The patient is then turned to the knee–chest position (Fig. 11.1) using knee resting supports and lithotomy poles to give support to the iliac crests. The head of the table is lowered by 15–20°. Clyman's self-retaining perineal retractor (Fig. 11.2) is inserted and a vulsellum is used to draw down the posterior lip of the cervix, thus

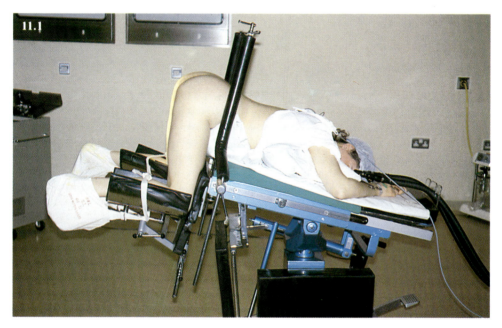

11.1

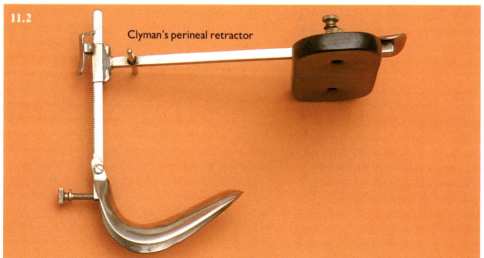

11.2 Clyman's perineal retractor

displaying the uterosacral ligaments which stand out as firm cords beneath the vaginal epithelium (Fig. 11.3). The dimple outlined between the ligaments indicates the puncture site (Fig. 11.4), which is infiltrated with 1% procaine and 1:200,000 adrenaline. The cervix is then pushed forwards towards the pubic symphysis, separating the walls of the pouch and placing the posterior fornix under tension. A Verres needle is inserted and the passage of air into the peritoneal cavity confirms a successful puncture. The opening is dilated with Hegar's dilators to allow insertion of a 4 or 8mm culdoscope (Fig. 11.5).

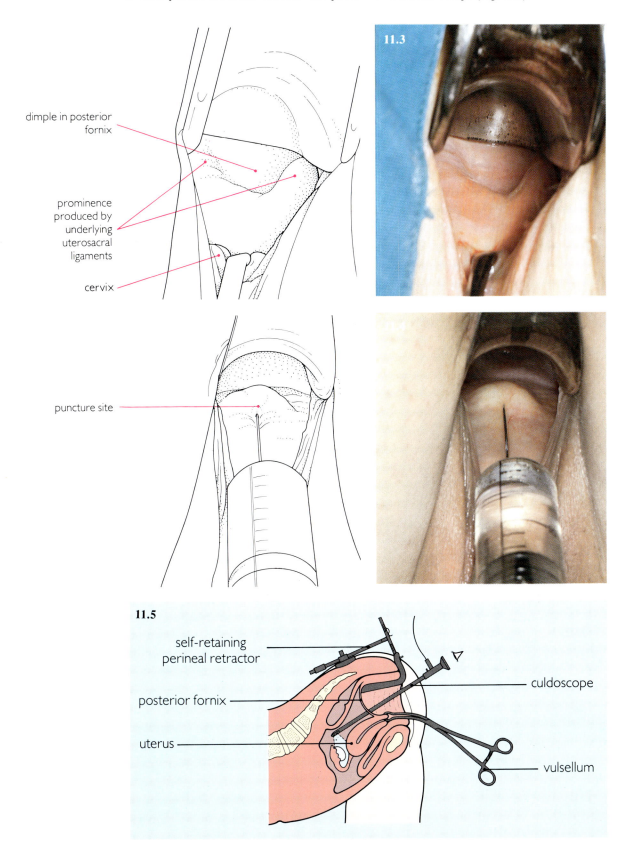

Normal findings

Culdoscopy allows a close-up view of the posterior surfaces of the uterus, ovaries and fimbriae of the tubes when the organs are in their natural positions (Fig. 11.6). By adjusting the cervical traction and pressing on the anterior abdominal wall, other aspects of the ovaries and tubes may be brought into view but the anterior wall of the uterus is not accessible.

In Fig. 11.7, the right ovary is clearly seen with the caecum in the background; if the telescope is brought nearer to the appendages, a closer view of the ovary and fimbriae is obtained (Fig. 11.8).

The upper abdominal cavity is not usually visible using the culdoscope, but it is possible to see the urachus and the lower anterior abdominal wall, as well as the uterine fundus,

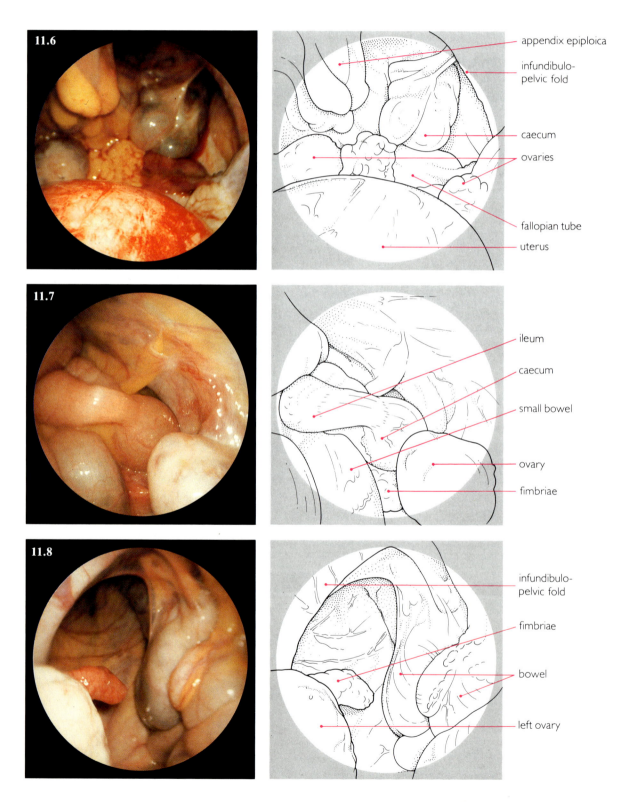

11.6
appendix epiploica
infundibulo-pelvic fold
caecum
ovaries
fallopian tube
uterus

11.7
ileum
caecum
small bowel
ovary
fimbriae

11.8
infundibulo-pelvic fold
fimbriae
bowel
left ovary

caecum and appendix (Fig. 11.9) providing the patient is not too obese.

Infertility

Investigation of infertility is one of the main indications for culdoscopy as the view obtained of the adnexa is usually excellent. A close-up view of the ovary in Fig. 11.10 shows a recently ruptured Graafian follicle with loops of bowel above the ovary; in Fig. 11.11 the ovary contains multiple follicular cysts.

When testing tubal patency, an 8 gauge Foley catheter with a 5ml balloon and the tip amputated is passed into the uterine cavity. During instillation of dye, the catheter is drawn gently downwards so that the balloon occludes outflow from the cervix. Patency can be demonstrated by hydropertubation with dilute

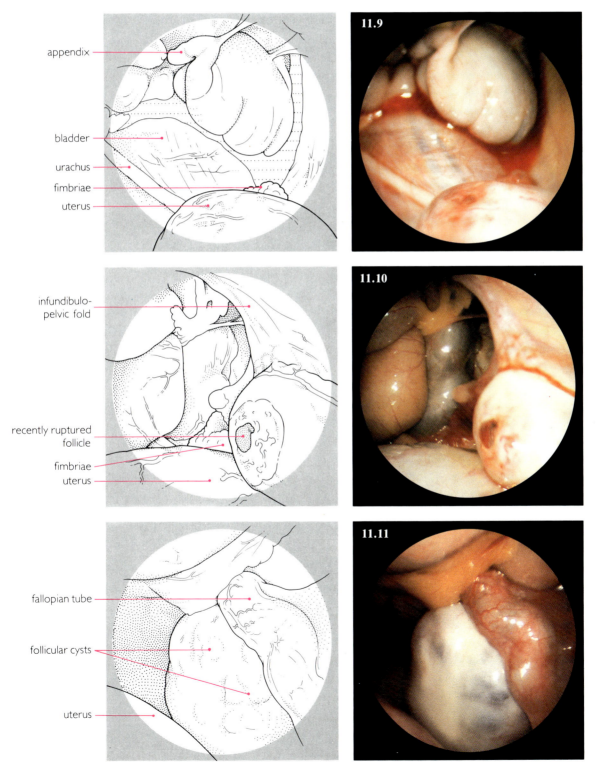

appendix

bladder

urachus

fimbriae

uterus

11.9

infundibulo-
pelvic fold

recently ruptured
follicle

fimbriae

uterus

11.10

fallopian tube

follicular cysts

uterus

11.11

indigo carmine. In panoramic view, the dye is seen accumulating in the pelvis if there is bilateral tubal patency (Fig. 11.12). When the telescope is advanced towards the tube, the dye is seen issuing from the fimbriae (Fig. 11.13). In Fig. 11.14, although the tube is patent, there are adhesions between the tube and ovary which are contributing to infertility; these will require microsurgical adhesiolysis to restore normal tubal function.

Abnormal findings
Several pathological lesions can be identified by culdoscopy. Fibroids, especially those on

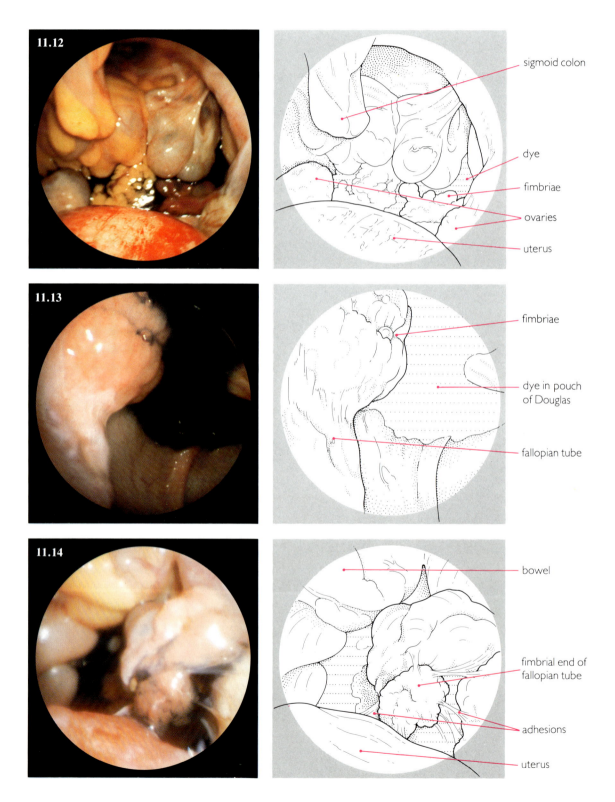

11.12

sigmoid colon
dye
fimbriae
ovaries
uterus

11.13

fimbriae
dye in pouch of Douglas
fallopian tube

11.14

bowel
fimbrial end of fallopian tube
adhesions
uterus

the posterior wall and uterine fundus (Fig. 11.15), are easy to see but those on the anterior wall are inaccessible. The ovaries are seen in detail and the advantage of culdoscopy over laparoscopy in this respect is that endometriosis can often be seen on the underside of the ovary (Fig. 11.16) without having to lift it up with a second instrument.

The sequelae of pelvic inflammatory disease also can be seen, although care must be taken because of the possibility of adhesions in the pouch of Douglas. Using the 'finger meeting' test will avoid accidental damage to adherent structures. In Fig. 11.17 a band of adhesions stretches from the appendix to the fundus of the uterus, hiding the right adnexa.

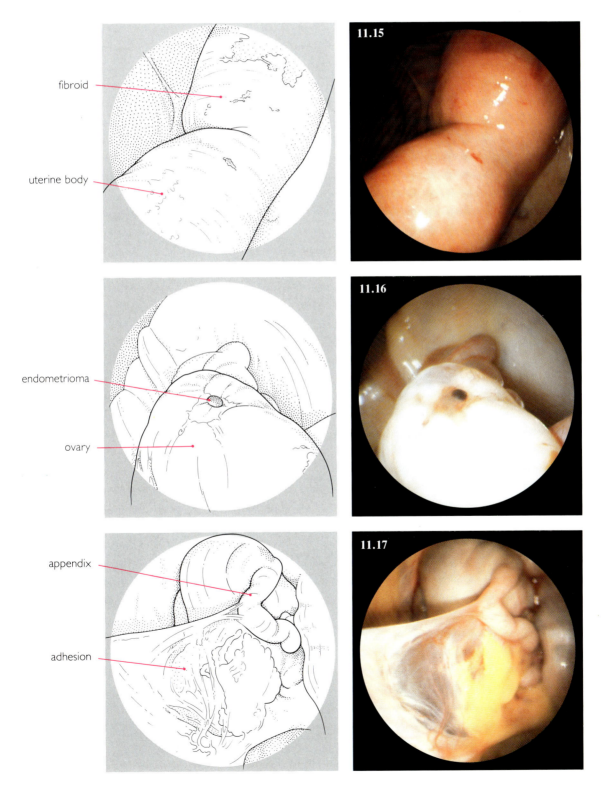

Tubal ligation

The introduction of operative instruments at culdoscopy allows oophorectomy, ovarian biopsy, division of adhesions and salpingostomy to be performed, but the most common culdoscopic operation is tubal ligation. The tube is first identified using the endoscope and the incision in the posterior fornix is extended transversely to 2–3cm (Fig. 11.18) using a diathermy knife; this controls any bleeding which would otherwise run down the telescope and obscure vision.

The tube is grasped with Clyman's clamp (Fig. 11.19), a double-angled light tissue clamp which enables the tube to be delivered into the

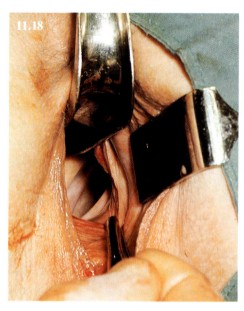
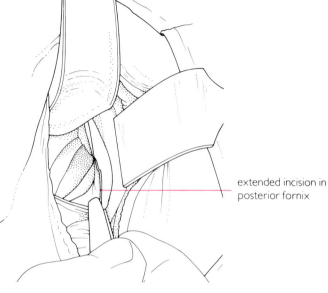

extended incision in posterior fornix

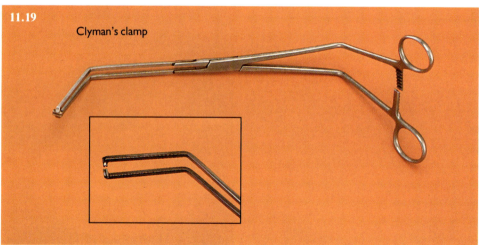

11.19 Clyman's clamp

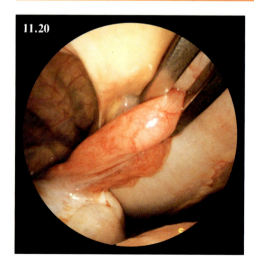
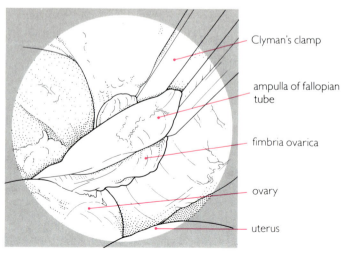

Clyman's clamp

ampulla of fallopian tube

fimbria ovarica

ovary

uterus

vagina. In Fig. 11.20 the ampulla is being held and the fimbriae are seen, with the fimbria ovarica attaching the tube to the ovary. Having identified the tube, the clamp is then repositioned to grasp the tubal isthmus (Fig. 11.21). If the tube is obscured by the ovary, the middle portion can be brought into view by simply pushing the ovary laterally with the tip of the clamp. Once the clamp has been applied, the culdoscope and vulsellum are removed and the loop of tube can usually be drawn into the vagina with gentle traction on the clamp (Fig. 11.22). A pair of curved artery forceps is then applied across the loop of tube produced by the clamp (Fig. 11.23), as in the Pomeroy method of tubal ligation.

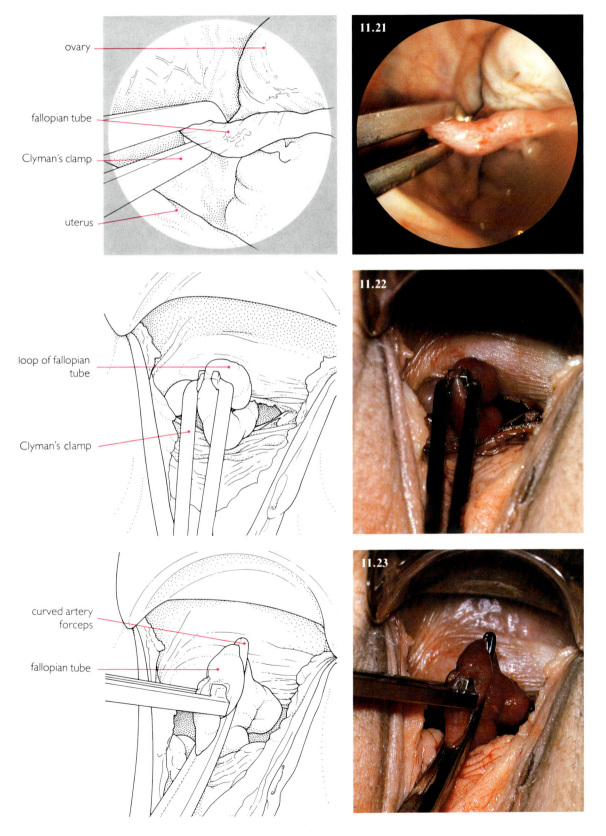

The apex of the loop of tube is excised with a knife (Fig. 11.24) and the cut ends ligated with catgut or Dexon (Fig. 11.25). This provides a section of tube for histological examination. Finally, the tube is inspected (Fig. 11.26) to ensure haemostasis before returning it to the abdominal cavity. On completion of culdoscopy, pressure is exerted on the abdominal wall by an assistant to expel air and the incision is closed with an absorbable suture. Some patients experience postoperative diaphragmatic irritation, which is relieved by assuming the supine position. Abstinence from intercourse is advised for two weeks following operative culdoscopy.

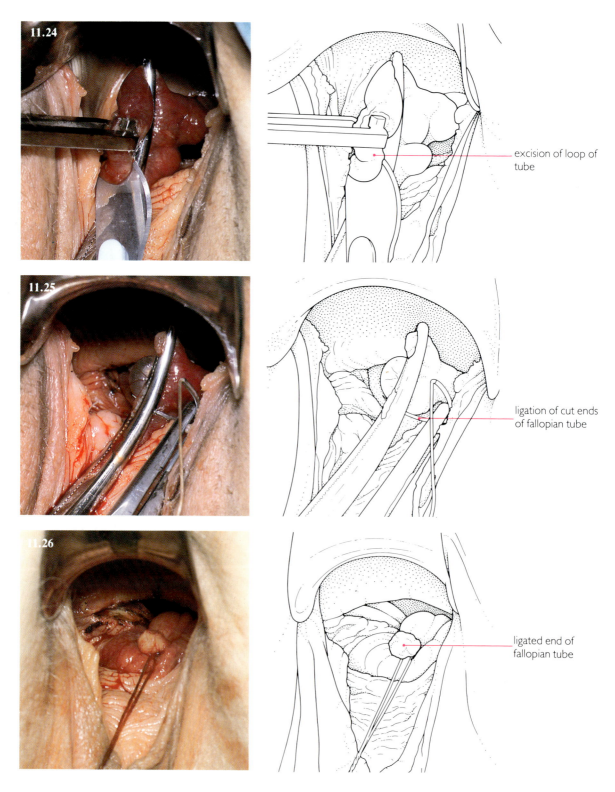

11.24

excision of loop of tube

11.25

ligation of cut ends of fallopian tube

11.26

ligated end of fallopian tube

12

IN VITRO FERTILIZATION

In vitro fertilization and embryo transfer are now becoming more widely available for the treatment of infertile couples. Infertility due to tubal blockage or adhesions, resulting from pelvic inflammatory disease, is conventionally treated by laparoscopic adhesiolysis or by salpingostomy using microsurgical techniques. If these approaches fail, IVF is preferable to additional surgery. When IVF was introduced by Steptoe and Edwards in 1978, treatment was restricted to women with irreparable tubal damage, but the indications have now been extended to include other conditions (Fig. 12.1) such as some cases of sperm motility defects and unexplained infertility, where there is no anatomical or physiological abnormality but conception has not occurred within two years.

Oocyte recovery
In each treatment cycle superovulation is induced because the pregnancy rate correlates with the number of embryos replaced, rising from about 10% with one embryo to 30% with three. If more than three embryos are replaced the risk of multiple pregnancy becomes unacceptably high. Most centres give clomiphene for five days followed by human menopausal gonadotrophin for up to six days, after which the dominant follicle should be ripe, as indicated by the rise in urinary oestrogen or the size of the follicle on ultrasound.

Oocyte recovery can be performed either laparoscopically or under ultrasound control. For laparoscopic recovery, one or both ovaries must be mobile and accessible; if this is not the case, preliminary adhesiolysis will be required. Most surgeons use a double-lumen needle (Fig.12.2), which is inserted into the follicle to aspirate the fluid; this is then examined by the embryologist using a phase contrast stereoscopic microscope. The follicle is repeatedly washed out with heparinized culture medium

12.1 Indications for in vitro fertilization

Bilateral tubal obstruction
cornual block gross hydrosalpinx post-sterilization
Bilateral salpingectomy
fimbriectomy
Extensive electrocoagulation
Extensive peritubal or periovarian adhesions
Extensive pelvic endometriosis
Sperm– mucus hostility
Oligospermia
Defective sperm motility
Unexplained infertility

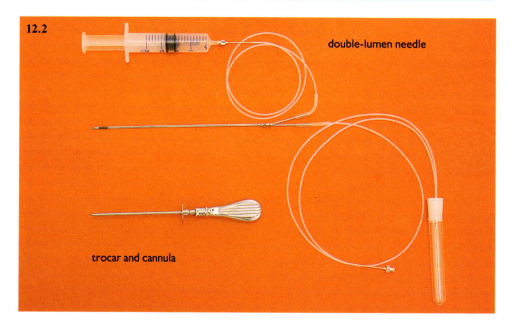
12.2 double-lumen needle; trocar and cannula

until an oocyte is identified. Some surgeons prefer to use single-lumen needles for both aspiration and flushing, as they feel that tearing of the follicle and leakage of fluid is less likely to occur with this than with a double-lumen needle. Suction can be provided simply by a syringe but is better applied using a foot-operated pump (Fig. 12.3), which produces a negative pressure of 60–100mm Hg.

The ovarian ligament is grasped with atraumatic holding forceps to bring the ovary into view and allow both sides of it to be examined. The dominant preovulatory follicle is easily recognized (Fig. 12.4) and the needle is inserted from the side (Fig. 12.5) rather than through its thinnest point. The follicle collapses when the fluid is aspirated (Fig. 12.6)

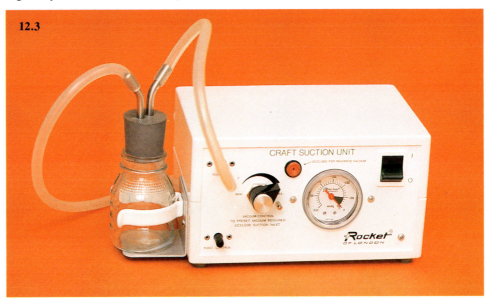

12.3

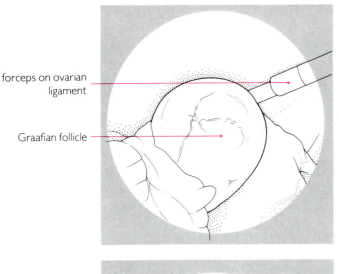

forceps on ovarian ligament

Graafian follicle

12.4

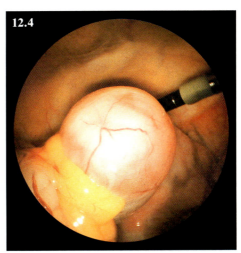

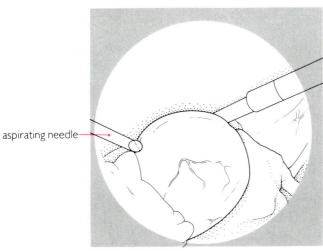

aspirating needle

12.5

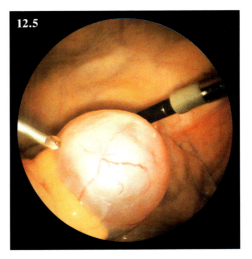

and repeated washing is then performed until the oocyte is obtained.

An alternative approach to laparoscopy is transvesical ultrasound-directed oocyte recovery (TUDOR). This is an outpatient technique performed under local anaesthesia. The bladder is first filled and the hyper-stimulated ovary is then visualized ultra-sonically (Fig. 12.7). A double-lumen needle is inserted through the abdominal wall and bladder into the follicle, and the oocyte is aspirated. The follicle collapses (Fig. 12.8) as the fluid is withdrawn.

This technique is especially useful if the ovary is fixed by dense adhesions and thus inaccessible to laparoscopy. A transvaginal approach can be used if the ovary is adherent in the pouch of Douglas. The procedure takes about 30–45 minutes. Complications are few, but there may be mild haematuria for a few hours afterwards. The patient can usually return home after a short rest.

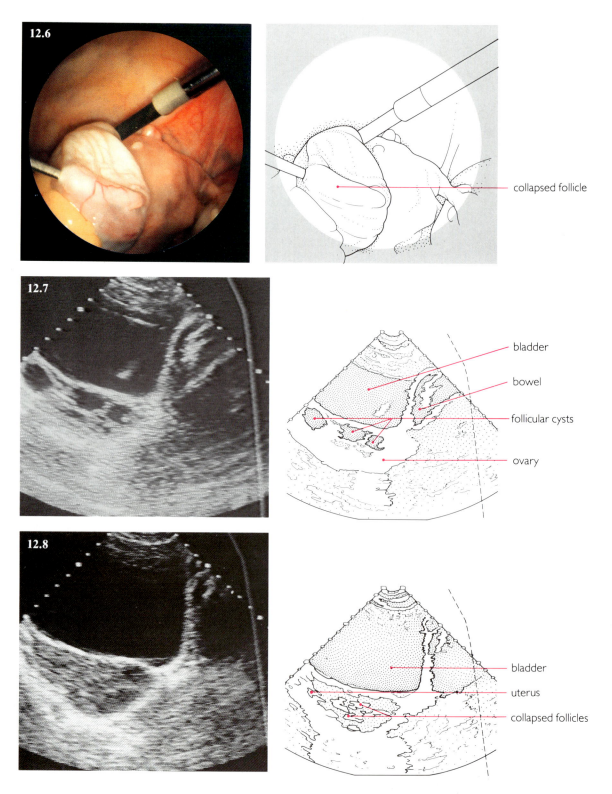

Fertilization

Successful fertilization can be recognized under the phase contrast microscope when the egg cleaves to produce first a two-cell and then a four-cell embryo (Fig. 12.9). There are numerous sperm outside the zona pellucida and a few granulosa cells are still present. Embryo transfer is usually performed at the four- or eight-cell stage (Fig. 12.10). The regular outline of each cell suggests normal development. By the time a morula has been formed by further cleavage divisions, it is probably too late for embryo transfer and degenerative changes (Fig. 12.11) and death of the embryo soon follow.

Embryo transfer

Embryo transfer is performed by inserting a fine Teflon catheter (Fig. 12.12) through the cleansed cervix. The inner lumen is preloaded with the embryos in 20–30μl of culture medium; if greater volumes are used, the

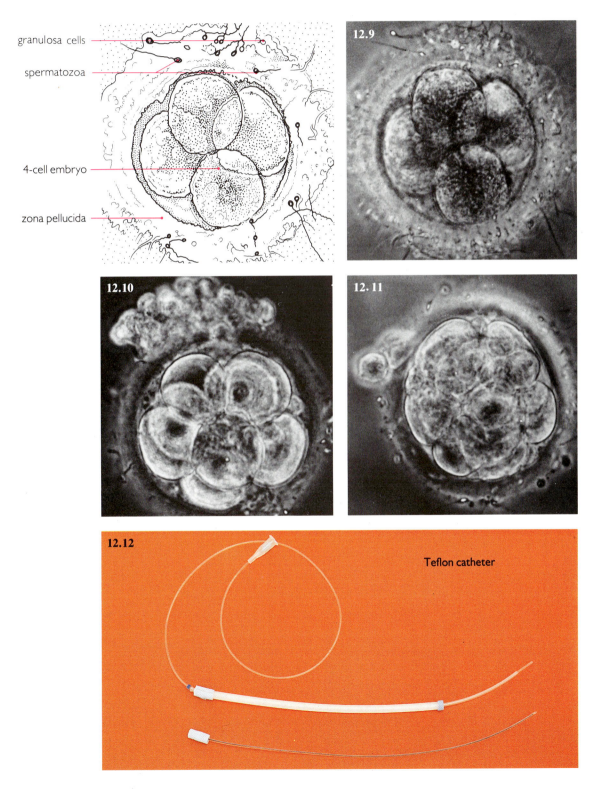

granulosa cells

spermatozoa

4-cell embryo

zona pellucida

12.9

12.10

12.11

12.12

Teflon catheter

embryos can be washed into the fallopian tubes with a risk of subsequent tubal pregnancy. Following transfer, the patient rests on her side with her hips elevated for a few hours before returning home. Beta-hCG measurements are performed ten days later to confirm implantation.

Gamete intrafallopian transfer

Gamete intrafallopian transfer (GIFT) is an alternative method in which the oocyte is obtained laparoscopically and then trans-ferred, together with washed sperms, via the fimbriae and into the fallopian tube by means of a small catheter (Fig. 12.13). Up to two oocytes with 100,000 sperms are instilled into each fallopian tube in a volume of $25\mu l$ of culture medium.

In young women with unexplained infertility and normal tubes, pregnancy rates of up to 40% have been reported following gamete intrafallopian transfer. This technique is also of value in patients with cervical mucus–sperm hostility.

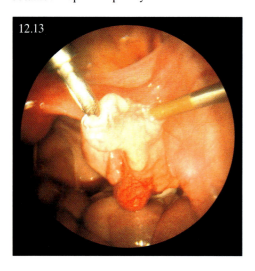

12.13

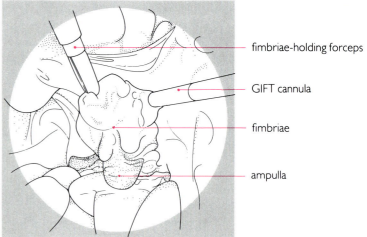

fimbriae-holding forceps

GIFT cannula

fimbriae

ampulla

CHAPTER

13

CHORIONOSCOPY

As a result of the dramatic fall in perinatal mortality in the western world, the importance of early recognition of congenital abnormalities has increased. Prenatal diagnosis of chromosome abnormalities and of some inborn errors of metabolism is now common obstetric practice. Transabdominal amniocentesis in patients at risk is not possible until at least the fifteenth week of gestation, whereas chorion villus biopsy can be performed from the ninth to the eleventh week. Biopsy of the chorion has a number of advantages. The tissue is fetal and is accessible during the first trimester by a transcervical or transabdominal approach. Furthermore, it can be obtained without perforating the fetal membranes and, since a diagnosis is available quickly, first trimester termination of pregnancy can be offered if necessary.

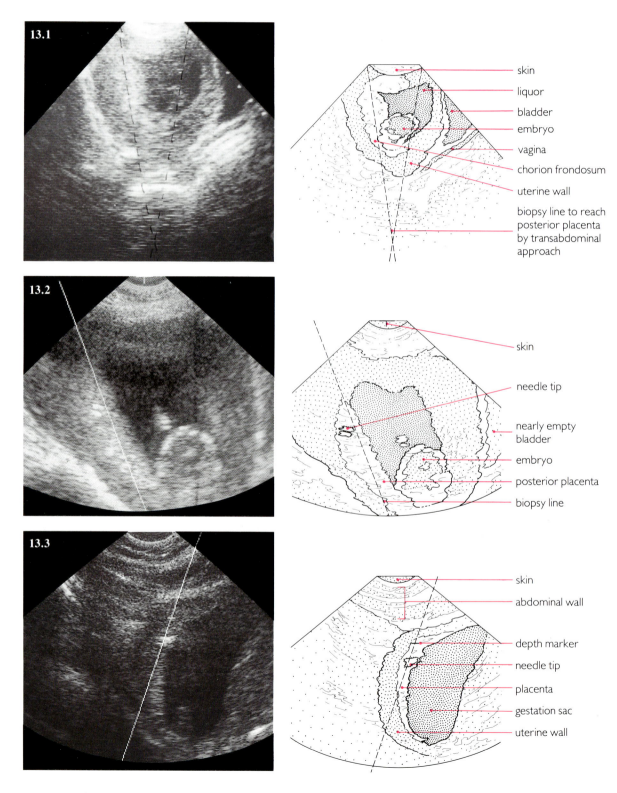

Biopsy under ultrasound control

Chorion villus biopsy was originally performed in China by blind transcervical aspiration of the villi to determine the sex of the fetus. The technique which is now used involves insertion of a malleable cannula through the cervix, guided by ultrasound; the villous tissue is obtained by aspiration using suction applied with a syringe. A more recent technique is the transabdominal transvesical approach shown in Figs.13.1–13.3, in which the aspirating needle is guided, under ultrasound control, through the bladder and into the chorion. The approach to the anterior uterine wall is usually easy but to gain access to chorion on the posterior wall, the bladder must be emptied to allow anteversion of the uterus.

Chorionoscopy

While ultrasound remains the method of choice, the newly developed technique of chorionoscopy allows easy examination of the villi in early pregnancy. The chorionoscope (Fig.13.4), developed by Ghirardini (1985), is a 4mm telescope with a small window and a villus-collecting chamber near its tip. The gestational age and placental site are determined by preliminary ultrasound. The chorionoscope, with its collecting chamber closed, is introduced through the cervix without anaesthesia; the chamber is then opened and the telescope advanced to the placental site.

A small volume of normal saline is injected through the syringe and side tube. This clears the visual field of blood and the villous fronds are seen floating in the fluid. The saline also magnifies the view in the same way as a drop on a slide does in microscopy. The villi are identified and aspirated into the collecting chamber, which is then closed to sever and retain them for examination.

This technique allows examination of the chorion in a retroverted uterus, when the placenta is posterior (Fig.13.5) and in obese patients, where examination by ultrasound may be difficult.

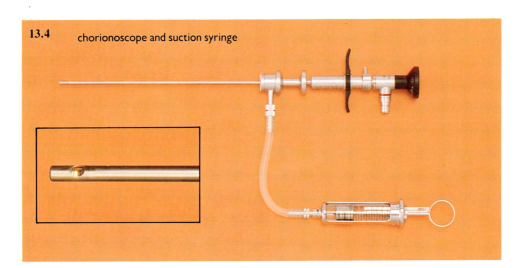

13.4   chorionoscope and suction syringe

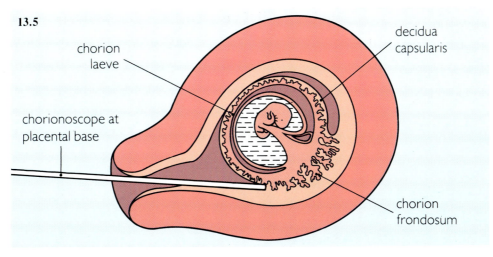

13.5

chorion laeve

chorionoscope at placental base

decidua capsularis

chorion frondosum

Chorionoscopy is only possible from the ninth to the thirteenth week of gestation; before this, the thickness of the decidua capsularis makes the investigation difficult. The clear view obtained allows the surgeon to distinguish the vascular villi of the chorion frondosum from the avascular villi of the chorion laeve.

A normal villus (Fig. 13.6) is vascular with a large number of syncytial sprouts; behind this, the smooth surface of the chorion and chorionic vessels can be seen. A large chorionic vessel in Fig. 13.7 is crossing the field of vision where, again, the villi are vascular and have numerous syncytial buds. Fig. 13.8 shows well vascularized villi in the chorion frondosum at slightly lower magnification.

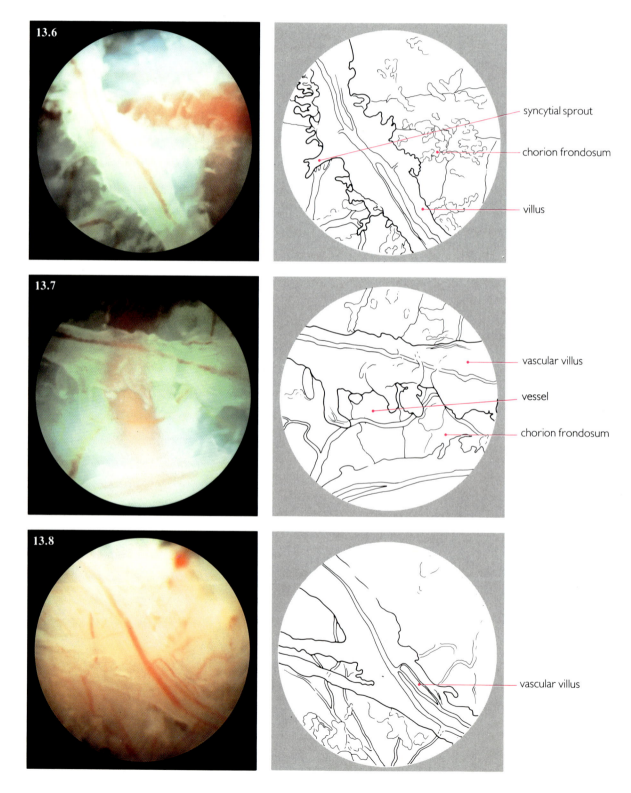

The number of syncytial sprouts and the vascularity of the villi show considerable variability. Fig. 13.9 shows the chorion frondosum with vascular villi, but they are smooth in outline and have only a few sprouts. As the telescope is moved away from the chorion frondosum towards the chorion laeve, a mixed picture, with both vascular and avascular villi (Fig.13.10), appears. Fig. 13.11 shows bleeding at the margin of the placental insertion in a patient with threatened abortion. The villi have buds but they are poorly vascularized.

Villi are present over the whole circumference of the early blastocyst but as it enlarges, it compresses the superficial decidua capsularis which becomes avascular. The villi

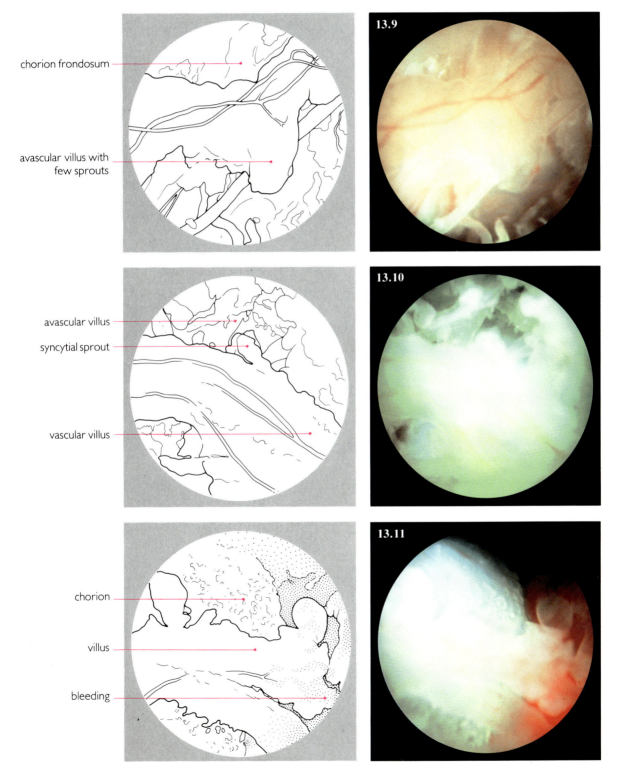

in the compressed part of the decidua capsularis atrophy and disappear and the surface of the chorion becomes smooth to form the chorion laeve. The villi over the surface of the early pregnancy sac are avascular (Fig. 13.12) and may be hydropic (Fig. 13.13). Fig. 13.14 shows anchoring villi in the chorion attaching it to the decidua.

Hysteroscopic biopsy

A hysteroscopic method of chorion villus biopsy has recently been developed by Van der Pas. This can be performed as early as the sixth week of pregnancy as an outpatient procedure, without anaesthesia. The uterus is distended with carbon dioxide, which is introduced at a flow rate of not more than 50ml/min; a higher

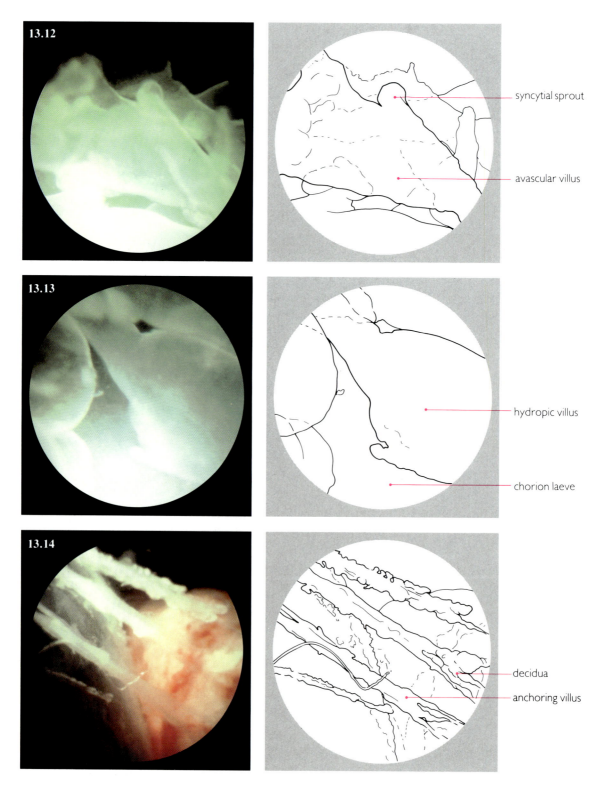

13.12 — syncytial sprout, avascular villus

13.13 — hydropic villus, chorion laeve

13.14 — decidua, anchoring villus

flow rate can cause the uterus to balloon and overdistend, introducing a possible danger of gas embolism.

The hysteroscope with operating sheath (Fig.13.15) is inserted. A cervical cap and handle allows control of the biopsy forceps and also enables the instrument to be held steady, an essential part of the procedure; this also leaves the operator's hand free to manipulate the biopsy forceps. The pregnancy sac is seen to protrude into the cavity (Fig.13.16), covered by the decidua capsularis. The vascular villi are accessible only when a window is cut in the decidua capsularis, near its junction with the decidua vera (Fig.13.17); thus the technique is difficult when the insertion is in the fundus.

Biopsy forceps are introduced along the operating channel of the hysteroscope and a

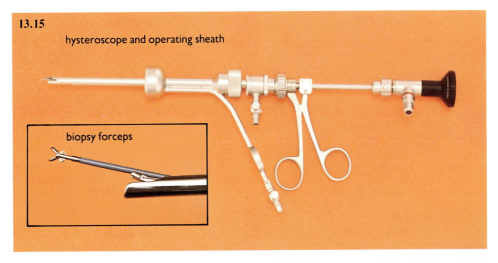

13.15

hysteroscope and operating sheath

biopsy forceps

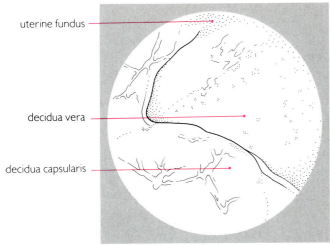

uterine fundus

decidua vera

decidua capsularis

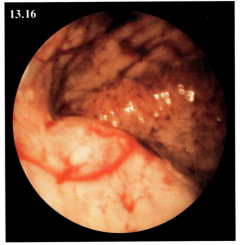

13.16

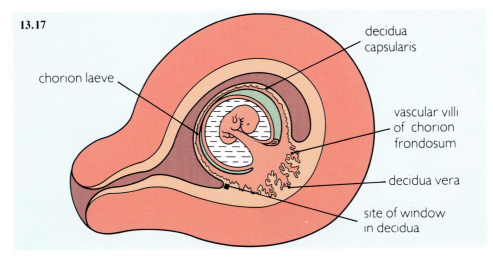

13.17

chorion laeve

decidua capsularis

vascular villi of chorion frondosum

decidua vera

site of window in decidua

small piece of decidua is removed, producing a window (Fig.13.18) which allows access to the underlying villi. The piece of decidua is discarded and the window enlarged if necessary. The telescope is gradually advanced (Fig.13.19) and, when close to the window (Fig.13.20), the chorion can be seen and a biopsy taken under direct vision. By repeating the biopsy, a sufficient amount of tissue can be obtained for chromosome analysis.

All methods of chorion villus biopsy carry a risk of producing bleeding and abortion; the risk is proportional to the skill and experience of the operator, but is not less than 2%.

Reference

Ghirardini G, Camurri L, Gualerzi C, Fochi F, Foscolu AMS, Spreafico L & Agnelli P (1985). In *First Trimester Fetal Diagnosis*. Edited by M.Fracaro. Berlin: Springer-Verlag.

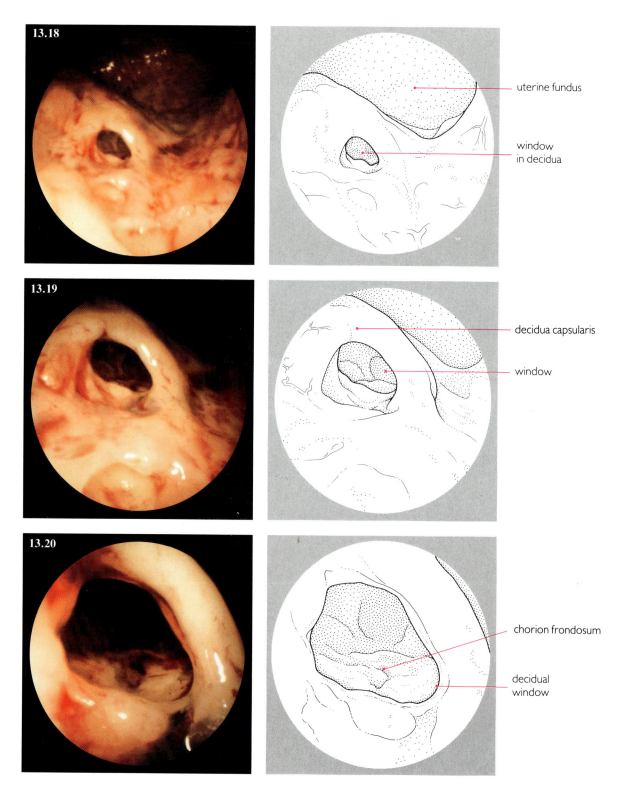

14

ANAESTHESIA AND ANALGESIA

I. F. RUSSELL

A. G. GORDON

Most gynaecological endoscopic procedures are of short duration, and so the anaesthetic techniques required are relatively simple. Nevertheless, these operations must be performed in a theatre which is fully equipped to deal with complications, both surgical and anaesthetic, as they occur. Some endoscopic techniques can be performed under local or regional anaesthesia, but in these cases the surgeon must bear in mind not only the possible surgical complications but also the toxicity of the analgesic and the dangers of accidental intravenous injection. An anaesthetist should always be available in the theatre in case of pain or complications requiring resuscitation or laparotomy.

Many endoscopic procedures can be performed on a day care basis, although pelviscopy is a major operation requiring several days in hospital. It must be accepted that a small percentage of day cases will experience pain or be unfit to go home and so facility must always be available for an overnight stay. The ability of the anaesthetist and surgeon to complete the operation within a reasonable time will dictate whether or not the patient can be treated as a day case; if the anaesthetic is over 30 minutes' duration, there is a greater chance of the patient having postoperative symptoms. The distance the patient lives from the hospital will also be a limiting factor, as she should not have a journey of more than one hour's duration on the same day as the operation.

General anaesthesia

Conventionally, general anaesthesia for laparoscopy entails the use of muscle relaxants, endotracheal intubation and assisted ventilation of the lungs. The major decision involved with this technique is the choice of muscle relaxant. Suxamethonium is widely used, but there is a high incidence of postoperative muscle pain. However, the recent introduction of atracurium and vecuronium, which are relatively short-acting, nondepolarizing muscle relaxants, has meant that suxamethonium can be replaced.

The advantages of intubation and assisted respiration (Fig.14.1) include a lax abdominal wall and controlled ventilation, which minimizes the respiratory effects of the pneumo-

14.1

Assisted and spontaneous respiration in general anaesthesia for laparoscopy		
	ADVANTAGES	DISADVANTAGES
Intubation and assisted respiration	Abdominal wall relaxed	Potential minor trauma
	No inhalation of gastric contents	
	Steep Trendelenburg possible	Longer induction and recovery time
	Duration not limited	
	Ventilation allows anaesthetist mobility	Complications of muscle relaxant
Spontaneous respiration	Reduced patient morbidity	Less abdominal muscle relaxation
	Simple induction and maintenance of anaesthesia	Limited Trendelenburg position

peritoneum, and the ability to use a steep Trendelenburg position. The anaesthetist is also free to respond immediately to any complication which might arise. The disadvantages of the technique include a higher morbidity related to the use of muscle relaxants and intubation, potential minor trauma such as sore throat, trauma to lips, teeth and gums, muscle pains if suxamethonium has been used, and the potentially disastrous failed intubation. This technique is also more time consuming, which may be an important factor in a busy operating list.

With increasing experience, laparoscopy becomes quicker and the volume of gas insufflated is reduced. There is thus less respiratory embarrassment, which reduces the need for controlled ventilation. Consequently, more laparoscopies are now being performed with patients breathing spontaneously through a mask, which confers several anaesthetic advantages. It is a simple, quick procedure with none of the morbidity associated with muscle relaxants, however, there is poor abdominal relaxation and possibly a restriction of the degree and duration of Trendelenburg position.

The choice of general anaesthetic technique will depend on the requirements and expertise of the operator, the expected duration of the procedure and the physical characteristics of the patient, such as obesity, expensive dental bridges and crowns and previous problems with intubation.

General anaesthesia for hysteroscopy is best administered by the simplest means possible and will usually involve the patient breathing spontaneously through a face mask, thus avoiding the use of muscle relaxants.

Local anaesthesia
Local anaesthesia for hysteroscopy is usually unnecessary if the cervix is patulous, but can be provided by bilateral paracervical block when the cervix is closed. It is advisable, on safety grounds, that an intravenous cannula should be in place before starting the block. A low concentration of local anaesthetic, such as 0.5% lignocaine in a dose of 5–8ml, should be injected into the vaginal fornix on each side at the 4 and 8 o'clock positions (Fig. 14.2). This blocks the pain fibres, innervating both the uterus and the cervix, from T10, T11, T12 and L1.

14.2

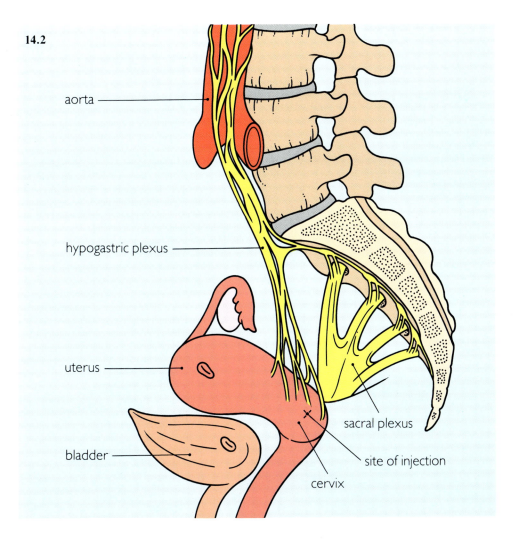

aorta

hypogastric plexus

uterus

bladder

sacral plexus

site of injection

cervix

Culdoscopy, although theoretically possible with local infiltration, is best performed under general anaesthesia with muscle relaxation, endotracheal intubation and artificial ventilation. The main difference between this and the procedure used for laparoscopy will be the position of the patient. Care is required to ensure a safe and stable position, with correct control of the patient's head, neck and arms during turning and positioning, while at the same time ensuring that the endotracheal tube is not displaced.

Local anaesthesia is suitable for a large proportion of patients having laparoscopic sterilization and for a smaller number undergoing other operations of short duration, such as investigation of pain or the suitability of the tubes for reversal of sterilization, but not for the investigation of infertility which demands a more detailed examination of the pelvis. The patient should be counselled pre-operatively and given 10mg of oral temazepam about one hour before going to theatre, where she receives 0.1mg of fentanyl intravenously.

As the patient is awake, the standard operating technique must be modified, using a Weisman–Graves speculum (Fig. 14.3) to insert the cervical tenaculum, the speculum being subsequently removed. The uterus can then be freely manipulated by the tenaculum without producing discomfort.

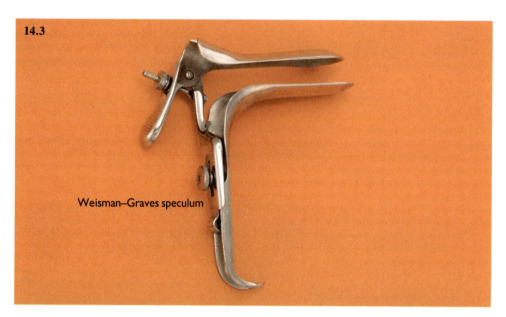

14.3

Weisman–Graves speculum

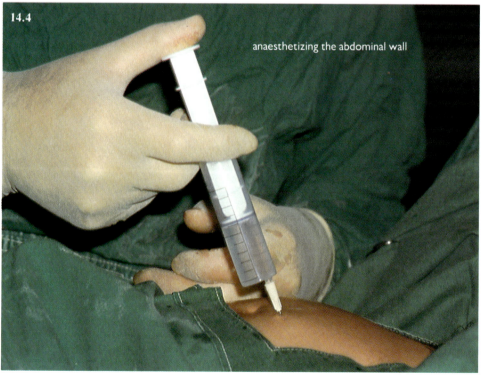

14.4

anaesthetizing the abdominal wall

The umbilicus and the site of the second incision are each infiltrated with 20ml of 0.5% lignocaine, ensuring that the full depth of the abdominal wall is anaesthetized. While the needle is being introduced (Fig. 14.4) and again, while the Verres needle (Fig. 14.5) and other instruments are being inserted, the patient is asked to push out her abdominal wall, giving a firm platform for the surgeon to push against. This manoeuvre also ensures that the abdominal wall is lifted away from the underlying vessels and organs. While inserting the trocar of the laparoscope (Fig. 14.6) it is important to hold one hand underneath the pushing hand to prevent sudden penetration and possible trauma. If the second puncture is made laterally through the rectus sheath, care must be taken to prevent the trocar skidding caudally on the surface of the sheath and penetrating the peritoneum at a distance from the site of the anaesthetic.

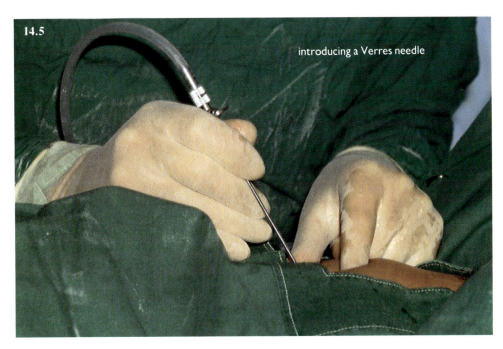

14.5   introducing a Verres needle

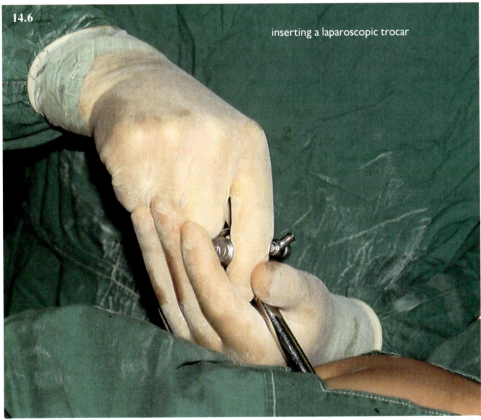

14.6   inserting a laparoscopic trocar

14.5

Whenever patients are under local anaesthesia the theatre staff must learn to work quietly and without verbal instruction. A quiet dialogue is conducted between the surgeon and the patient as each step of the operation is explained.

Laparoscopy under local anaesthesia should not be considered if the patient has any fears about the operation. Obesity is not a contraindication provided the abdominal wall is not too thick, but any suspicion of intra-abdominal adhesions should be an indication for general anaesthesia.

In the majority of patients the operation is completely acceptable. Some pain occurs in about 3% of patients but it is rarely severe. Pain may be caused by the pneumoperitoneum, or may be due to incomplete anaesthesia of the abdominal wall. Compression of the tubes by clips or rings also produces pain, but rarely interferes with successful completion of the operation.

15

PHOTOGRAPHY

Endoscopic photography is becoming an essential skill in gynaecological practice. It is vital for accurate documentation of operative findings, as no description or line drawing conveys information so accurately as a photograph. It is valuable in assessing the results of treatment of malignant disease, endometriosis and operations for infertility, and is also of use in documenting tubal sterilization for legal purposes. Counselling patients about planned operations and obtaining 'informed consent' are greatly assisted by the use of photographs.

In medical education and training of resident staff, it is essential to have a range of photographic slides to illustrate the normal and abnormal anatomy, which may not be available for demonstration in theatre.

The standard light source is not bright enough for still photography so an electronic flash is necessary. Originally, the flash bulb was incorporated in the distal end of the telescope, but this was dangerous and could cause burns and electric shock. The modern proximal electronic flash unit (Fig. 15.1) eliminates this risk because the light is transmitted to the telescope via a fibreoptic or liquid cable. In the fully automatic version, the exposure time is calculated electronically.

In the majority of cases, the camera used is an automatic 35mm single lens reflex (SLR) model with a special focusing screen for endoscopic work. Most cameras have this ability but only a few, such as the Olympus OM-1 or OM-2, have readily interchangeable screens. The camera is attached to the eyepiece of the telescope by an adaptor lens with a 90mm focal length. By increasing the focal length to 140mm, the image takes up more of the screen and the circular format is altered to a rectangular one (Fig. 15.2).

Most medical photographers use 35mm reversible film for transparencies rather than print film because the definition is better. If the film is too fast the results will show increased grain and definition will be poor, so film with a speed (ASA) of 200–400 is preferable. Polaroid have produced an instant slide film, but with an ASA of 40 it is too slow for most light sources.

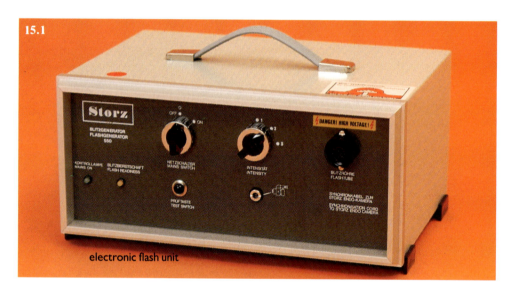

15.1

electronic flash unit

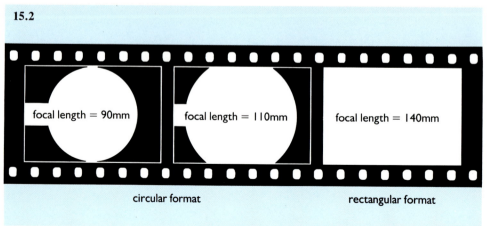

15.2

focal length = 90mm focal length = 110mm focal length = 140mm

circular format rectangular format

Whenever possible, a telescope with a large diameter should be used. For high quality laparoscopic work, a 10 or 11mm instrument is necessary but in other endoscopic procedures such a large lens is impracticable.

A system less commonly used is the Olympus 16mm camera, which is small and lightweight and uses a cassette film. This is convenient but requires special projection equipment. The Polaroid instant camera system has endoscopic adaptors to provide prints for inclusion in the patient's notes. This is convenient but the quality is not good enough for publication, although it is adequate for documentation.

Endoscopic cinematography has been used in the past, but its application has now been superceded by closed-circuit colour television (CCTV). The systems available vary from a simple light source, camera and monitor (Fig. 15.3) to a complex system with a computer and word processor to annotate and provide a complete video documentation system (Fig. 15.4). The value of CCTV in theatre is that it is always available to demonstrate and record pathology for teaching purposes but, even more important, it allows supervision of staff being trained to undertake more complicated endoscopic procedures. It also allows them to assist at operations, holding instruments and retracting tissues.

The camera is usually attached to the laparoscope using a beam splitter, so that the surgeon can view the operation site directly

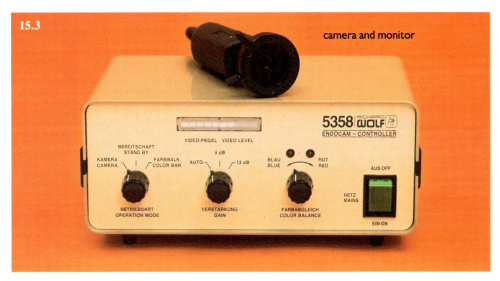

15.3   camera and monitor

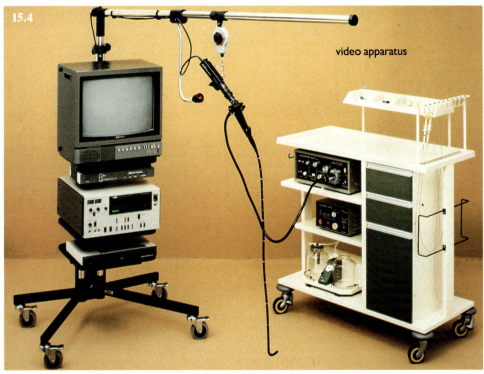

15.4   video apparatus

while assistants watch the monitor. In video-laparoscopy, the camera is directly attached to the telescope and the surgeon also watches the television screen. The tube camera (Fig. 15.5) is too heavy to be held for a long period of time by the operator and so should be held either by an assistant or by a counterbalanced arm, allowing it to be effectively weightless. A small chip camera (Fig. 15.6) is very light and thus ideal for videolaparoscopy. The quality and colour of the picture can be adjusted manually using the colour-control apparatus.

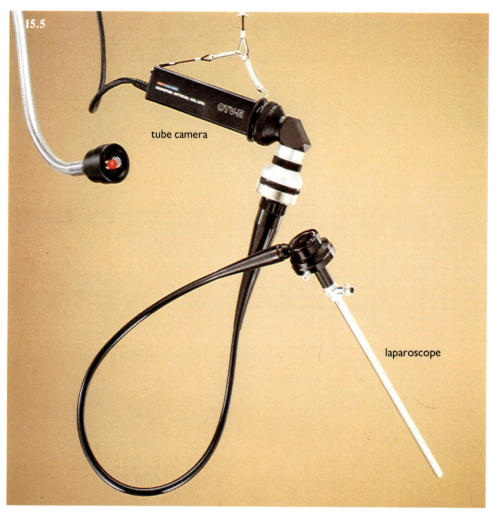

15.5 tube camera

laparoscope

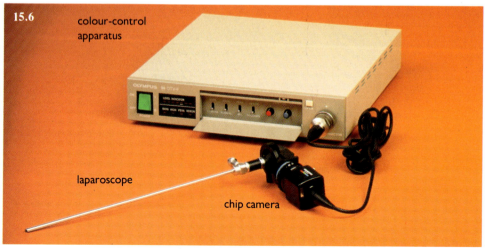

15.6 colour-control apparatus

laparoscope

chip camera

SOURCES OF TRANSPARENCIES

Chapter 2 Instruments for Endoscopy
Fig. 2.1-2.24 G I Whitehead

Chaper 3 Laparoscopy
Figs. 3.1-3.3 G I Whitehead
Fig. 3.4 H Frangenheim
Figs. 3.5-3.6 G I Whitehead
Fig. 3.7 B V Lewis
Fig. 3.8 A G Gordon
Figs. 3.9-3.10 B V Lewis
Fig. 3.11 A G Gordon
Fig. 3.12 A Auderbert
Fig. 3.13. K Semm
Fig. 3.14 B V Lewis
Figs. 3.15-3.18 A G Gordon
Figs. 3.19-3.21 B V Lewis
Fig. 3.22 A G Gordon
Fig. 3.23 G I Whitehead
Figs. 3.24-3.25 M Cognat
Fig. 3.27 B V Lewis
Fig. 3.28 H Frangenheim
Fig. 3.29 A Auderbert
Figs. 3.30-3.32 K Semm
Figs. 3.33-3.34 H J Lindemann
Fig. 3.35 H Frangenheim

Chapter 4 Infertility
Fig. 4.1 H Frangenheim
Fig. 4.2 B V Lewis
Fig. 4.3 A G Gordon
Fig. 4.4 H Frangenheim
Fig. 4.5 M R Darling
Fig. 4.6 A Auderbert
Fig. 4.7 H Frangenheim
Fig. 4.8 M Cognat
Figs. 4.9-4.12 H Frangenheim
Fig. 4.13 M R Darling
Fig. 4.14 K Semm
Fig. 4.15 H Frangenheim
Figs. 4.16-4.17 M Darling
Fig. 4.18 K Semm
Fig. 4.19 M Cognat
Fig. 4.20 M R Darling
Figs. 4.21-4.22 M Cognat
Fig. 4.23 H Frangenheim
Fig. 4.24 A G Gordon
Fig. 4.25 M Darling
Fig. 4.26 B V Lewis
Fig. 4.27 A Auderbert
Fig. 4.28 H Frangenheim
Figs. 4.29-4.31 K Semm
Fig. 4.32 M Cognat
Figs. 4.33-4.35 A Auderbert
Fig. 4.36 L Pous-Ivern
Figs. 4.37-4.38 A Auderbert
Fig. 4.39 B Hibbard
Fig. 4.40 A Auderbert
Fig. 4.41 B V Lewis
Fig. 4.42 H Frangenheim
Fig. 4.43 A Auderbert
Fig. 4.44 H Frangenheim
Fig. 4.45 A G Gordon
Fig. 4.46 H Frangenheim
Figs. 4.47-4.48 M Cognat
Fig. 4.49 H Frangenheim
Fig. 4.50 M Cognat
Figs. 4.51-4.52 H Frangenheim
Fig. 4.53 L Pous-Ivern

Fig. 4.54 M R Darling
Figs. 4.55-4.57 H Frangenheim
Fig. 4.58 B V Lewis
Fig. 4.59 M Cognat
Fig. 4.60 A Auderbert
Figs. 4.7-4.12 K Semm
Figs. 4.13-4.15 H Frangenheim

Chapter 5 Pelvic Inflammatory Disease
Figs 5.1-5.2 H Frangenheim
Fig. 5.3 B Hibbard
Fig. 5.4 H Frangenheim
Fig. 5.5 K Semm
Fig. 5.6 H Frangenheim
Figs. 5.7-6.10 A G Gordon
Fig. 5.11 B V Lewis
Fig. 5.12 A Auderbert
Figs. 5.13-5.17 C J G Sutton
Fig. 5.18 H Frangenheim
Figs. 5.19-5.20 K Semm
Fig. 5.21 A G Gordon
Fig. 5.22 H Frangenheim
Fig. 5.23 J S Scott
Fig. 5.24 H Frangenheim
Fig. 5.25 M Cognat
Fig. 5.26 L Pous-Ivern
Fig. 5.27 B Hibbard
Fig. 5.28 H Frangenheim
Fig. 5.29 A Auderbert
Figs. 5.30-5.32 H Frangenheim
Fig. 5.33 A G Gordon
Figs. 5.34-5.37 H Frangenheim
Fig. 5.38 A Auderbert
Fig. 5.39 B V Lewis
Fig. 5.40 A Auderbert
Fig. 5.41 H Frangenheim

Chapter 6 Endometriosis and Pelvic Pain
Fig. 6.1 A G Gordon
Figs. 6.2-6.3 L Pous-Ivern
Fig. 6.4 H Frangenheim
Fig. 6.5 B V Lewis
Fig. 6.6 A Auderbert
Figs. 6.7-6.9 H Frangenheim
Fig. 6.10 B V Lewis
Figs. 6.11-6.12 C J G Sutton
Figs. 6.13-6.15 H Frangenheim
Fig. 6.16 A Auderbert
Fig. 6.17 L Pous-Ivern
Fig. 6.18 B V Lewis
Figs. 6.19-6.20 A Auderbert
Fig. 6.21 B V Hibbard
Fig. 6.22 L Pous-Ivern
Fig. 6.23 H Frangenheim
Fig. 6.24 L Pous-Ivern
Fig. 6.25 H Frangenheim
Fig. 6.26 M Cognat
Figs. 6.27-6.29 K Semm
Fig. 6.30 B V Lewis
Fig. 6.31 B Hibbard
Fig. 6.32 A G Gordon
Fig. 6.33 K Semm
Fig. 6.34 H Frangenheim
Figs. 6.33-6.36 K Semm
Figs. 6.37-6.38 B V Lewis
Fig. 6.39 H Frangenheim
Fig. 6.40 M R Darling
Fig. 6.41 B V Lewis

INDEX

All entries refer to page numbers